THE

Insta-Food
DIET

ALSO BY PIXIE TURNER

The Wellness Rebel
Pixie's Plates
The No Need To Diet Book

THE
Insta-Food
DIET

PIXIE TURNER

HEAD
of ZEUS

An Anima Book

This is an Anima book, first published in the UK in 2020 by
Head of Zeus Ltd

9 7 5 3 1 2 4 6 8

A catalogue record for this book is available from
the British Library.

ISBN (HB): 9781788547185
ISBN (E): 9781788547208

Printed and bound in Great Britain by
CPI Group (UK) Ltd, Croydon CRO 4YY

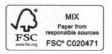

Head of Zeus Ltd
5–8 Hardwick Street
London EC1R 4RG

WWW.HEADOFZEUS.COM

CONTENTS

For my father, who loved food and didn't really get the whole social media thing.

INTRODUCTION

The very first food picture I posted on Instagram was taken back in 2012. It featured a salad bowl with a heavy filter, terrible yellow lighting and harsh shadows; it received very little attention or praise. Since then, I have posted thousands of food pictures online, and deleted several hundred along the way. Some tasted so awful I couldn't eat them, some were dishes other people had ordered, some were 'bulked up' to give the illusion of quantity, some were aesthetically pleasing yet boring, and others were incredibly delicious and attractive. Many gained me hundreds of new followers, and one or two have lost me several thousand followers overnight. Food is an incredibly polarising topic, and social media has given each of us huge power to use and abuse this.

I've been posting about food on social media for over eight years now. During my first year my account was private, then I found #cleancating and created a public wellness account that gained me over 80,000 followers in the space of two years. After that, I turned my back on the obsessive cult of Instagram wellness, and since 2015 I have been using my platforms as a tool for science communication.

The twenty-first century marked the emergence and growth of social networking sites that have since become a major part of people's lives. Few of us can imagine life without social media anymore, and it's unrealistic to assume that it's even possible.

There is a clear and growing body of research pointing to a link between social media use and mental health issues including depression, anxiety and eating disorders. We are starting to become more aware of the negative implications of social media, but we struggle to really accept these implications because in the immediate moment when we go online it lifts our mood. The negative effects come with more prolonged use.

Anyone who says getting likes and comments on their posts doesn't make them feel good is probably lying. It's a little dopamine hit that validates you as a person. In one study, the number of likes individuals received on their Facebook profile pictures was linked with higher self-esteem. But it's short-lived. In a survey in 2017, 89% of social media users said that getting plenty of likes on their pictures and posts makes them feel happy, but for 40% of them the happiness stops when the likes do. Only around 10% of people will carry that happiness for the whole day.

Social media may have had a huge effect on society – it's here now and it's here to stay – but something that was supposed to be fun has, for many of us, turned into a source of stress and anxiety. And yet so few of us are able and willing to step away from it. We say, 'I wish I could stop scrolling', clearly expressing a desire at least to reduce our time online, and yet we feel unable to do so.

Why is that? Well there's a clear answer: social media is where everyone is.

Everybody is online

In case it isn't clear: in this book, I will be using 'social media' to describe the platforms of Facebook, Twitter, Instagram, Pinterest and YouTube. Blogs will get a mention too. These are platforms that allow users to create personal profiles, form connections and communicate with others, create and share content, and access searchable online content posted by others. They are also the biggest social media platforms out there. Facebook is the largest with over 2 billion users, YouTube has 1.9 billion and Instagram just over 1 billion. In total, there were 3.48 billion social media users in 2019 – that's a lot of people. In fact, that equates to around 45% of the current world population.

Categorised by age, 48.2% of baby boomers, 77.5% of Generation X and 90.4% of millennials (Generation Y), are active social media users. Gen Z is likely just as high – if not higher – than millennials once age restrictions are taken into account.*

Social media isn't only impressive in terms of overall users, but it's startling just how much time we spend using them. Platforms such as Facebook, Instagram and Twitter have become ubiquitous, occupying 2 out of every 5 minutes we spend online. Among people aged 16–34, 60% feel they use their phone too much, with an average of 35% across all age groups. So, clearly, many of us realise we're spending too much time online, which is good news. The bad news is that we are not managing to moderate our use effectively. Only 14% of people who are trying to control their usage feel they are successfully doing so, and

---

* The age limit for most/all social media platforms is set to 13+.

most are taking no steps at all, despite explicitly stating they would like to.

Can we call social media addictive? Let's look at some of the stats:

* The average person spends 158 minutes per day on social media, which is around a third of their total Internet time.
* The average mobile phone user touches their phone 2,617 times per day, with the top 10% touching their phone 5,427 times.
* Data by Apple shows that the average user with Touch ID unlocks their iPhone every 11 minutes and 15 seconds.

OK, it's still clear we're using our phones a little too much perhaps. But is it addictive? Here are some more stats:

* 75% of smartphone users admit to using their phones while on the toilet, whether out of boredom or because they can't bear to part from it.
* 45% feel they need to constantly check their phone, or are distracted by their phone while completing a task.
* In 2011, a survey stated that 53% of young people aged 16–22 would rather lose their sense of smell than lose access to their phone or a computer.
* 79% of millennials keep their phones by their bed or even in their bed while they sleep, and more than half check their phone during the night.

Now this is starting to look a little more concerning. At this point I want to point out that it's easy to think this doesn't apply to us, that we're definitely on the low end of that. And you might be. But I challenge you, just for a day, to track how many times you pick up your phone, unlock it, stare at it and scroll – most phones let you view daily screen time, and the results may surprise you.

Looking at those stats you might immediately think 'yep, social media is definitely addictive', but it's worth digging a little deeper and examining both sides.

To those in camp 'Definitely Addictive', the answer is clear. Tech insiders have admitted that social media apps are specifically designed to exploit the reward system in our brains in order to keep us scrolling. Some have termed this 'brain hacking'. Sean Parker, who joined Facebook when it was just five months old, claimed in a 2017 interview with *Axios* that social media was designed to "consume as much of your time and conscious attention as possible". When the creators themselves are using this language, surely it must have been intended to be an addictive activity?

How many times have you seen a notification appear on your phone and immediately felt compelled to find out what it is? How often have you opened an app just to have a quick look, and then 20 minutes later you're still scrolling and reading? Do you feel the need to check all your social media apps systematically rather than stopping at just one? I do. First thing in the morning I start with emails (just viewing, not sending), then Twitter, followed by Facebook and ending on Instagram. Every morning. I do all of these things, and it feels automatic.

The 'like' button didn't exist in the first incarnation of Facebook, it was added later in 2009. It's hard to imagine Facebook without a 'like' button, it's such a key part of our interactions online. In fact, it's now so widely used that collectively we 'like' things 4.5 billion times each day. The Facebook engineer who created the 'like' button in the first place describes them as "bright dings of pseudo-pleasure". The idea behind it was to send "little bits of positivity" throughout the platform, and it was hugely successful. People's engagement with Facebook increased dramatically following its introduction, and it gave Facebook valuable data about our likes and dislikes, which can be sold to advertisers. The idea was such a success it's since been adopted by Twitter in the form of the 'heart' button, and by Instagram, again as a heart – 'double tap to like!'

For an app, generating more users isn't good enough anymore: they want loyal ones. Finding ways to get users to spend more time on social media means more ad revenue and more profit for these companies. Of course they want to keep you hooked.

Nir Eyal's bestselling 2014 book, *Hooked: How to Build Habit-Forming Products*, details the mechanism by which these apps capture our attention and vast swathes of our time. His Hook model includes several phases: trigger, action, reward and investment.

A trigger tells us what to do, for example 'click here!' On social media, the trigger is simply the icon, often with a little red circle* indicating the number of notifications we have. Through repeated exposure to these triggers, we start to develop associations between the trigger and our emotions or behaviours. If we open Twitter every time we're bored or scroll through Instagram when we're sad, we start to develop a habit of checking those platforms whenever those same feelings come up.

---

*   Red being the colour suggesting 'warning' or 'danger', which we then want to remove.

The action phase is simple: if there's enough motivation and the action is easy enough to do, it happens, and we respond to the trigger. Simply tapping on an icon on, say, your phone, is incredibly easy. The easier the action, the less motivation we need to muster to perform it.

The reward phase creates wanting through anticipation. Rewards on social media are incredibly variable – some posts will be interesting to you, while others are boring. However, what keeps you going is the anticipation that just a short scroll away you may find a post that intrigues you. Before you know it, half an hour has passed and you're still scrolling. In addition, those who post content are rewarded as much as their viewers, because social media also rewards you by showing you likes, comments, and follows/subscribers.

Within this process, anticipation of reward produces a dopamine hit in your brain. In an evolutionary context, it rewards us for beneficial behaviours and motivates us to repeat them. The neurotransmitter dopamine is associated with all things pleasurable and beneficial: food, exercise, love, sex, gambling, drugs... and now, social media. The anticipation of these pleasures increases the level of dopamine in the brain. When the rewards we anticipate are delivered to us at random, not consistently, we will keep pushing that trigger until it becomes a habit. This happens with slot machines where you don't know whether this next go is the one that'll give you the jackpot, or with social media where you don't know when or how many likes you will get.

The investment phase is arguably the most important as it requires some user input with the anticipation of longer-term rewards, not just instant gratification. For example, on Twitter or Instagram this occurs when you follow someone new and their posts start to appear on your timeline. You don't get a reward for following someone, but their content will keep you checking the app to see if they've posted anything since last time. You're now invested and come back daily to see what's new.

These apps also work through reciprocity: when you invest, they give you something back. Twitter allows you to view every tweet you've liked; on Facebook everything you share can be viewed by your friends; and Instagram has a feed dedicated to all the images you've been tagged in. The more time you invest in these apps and the more content you like and share, the more the algorithm curates your feed according to what you like to see, making you even more likely to engage. Rather than show you content in reverse chronological order, social media algorithms are a way of sorting posts in your feed based on what is mathematically deemed to be relevant to you, based on what you've engaged with in the past.* In this way, your investment is intended to enhance your experience. All these are examples of online content as stored value, and they make the next trigger more engaging than before. It also creates a barrier to you deleting your account, as all that time you've invested and the data you've input would disappear.

Arguably anything that produces a pleasurable sensation and gives you a dopamine hit has the potential to become addictive, but just because we could be using such language doesn't mean we should.

Interestingly, Nir Eyal doesn't agree with calling social media

---

* On Twitter and Facebook, you can still select between 'show me the best tweets first' or 'top stories', respectively, and 'newest first'. Instagram has no such option, and this is still something that pisses off a lot of people.

apps and sites addictive. His argument is that using addiction language creates a sense of 'learned helplessness'. According to the American Psychological Association, this occurs when someone repeatedly faces uncontrollable, stressful situations. They learn that they are helpless in that situation, and then when change is possible – when there's a chance for escape – they don't take it.

While this phrase is usually applied in the context of post-traumatic stress disorder (PTSD), it's also applicable to our social media use: if we're taught that these companies are 'hacking our brains' and we feel we have no control or power when it comes to these apps, we feel helpless and don't bother trying to change anything because what's the point? It's not possible anyway.

Clearly, I wouldn't be writing this book if I believed we had no real power to do anything, and experts generally agree with me, although you won't read much of this kind of narrative online because it doesn't generate clicks and sales in the same way as sensationalised catastrophising headlines do. We are not simply puppets on a string controlled by Facebook. We do have some power.

These ideas make you think: when we talk about social media, do we mean addiction or habit?

I don't sit on the fence about many topics, but this is one I find tricky. On the one hand, we have these apps, whose inventors and creators have explicitly stated were built to be as engaging as possible. This is understandable: after all, why would you create something that isn't engaging? We don't get angry at Netflix for making binge-worthy series that we just can't get enough of – we expect that. On the other hand, I recognise that calling social media 'addictive' can contribute to learned helplessness, and can leave people feeling that there's no point in even trying to reduce their consumption, which isn't exactly helpful. Here are some comparisons that show you the difference between addiction and habit. I'll leave you to make up your own mind.

	ADDICTION	HABIT
Definition	Repeated use of a substance or activity despite the negative consequences suffered by the addicted individual.	Automatic behaviours that we do with little to no conscious thought.
Conditions	Salience – has a significant or notable impact. Euphoria – activates pleasure and reward centres in the brain. Tolerance – such that more and more is needed to produce the same effect. Withdrawal symptoms – through lack of use. Conflict – interfering with other everyday activities and relationships. Relapse – despite efforts to reduce/avoid addictive substance.	Automatic – done often without awareness until pointed out by someone. Repetition – usually through association with a particular emotion, time or place. Lack of pleasure – often neither pleasurable nor painful.
Offline examples	Alcohol. Drugs.	Nail-biting. Walking the same route to the same bus stop.
Harmful?	Yes – addiction is a pathology.	Usually no.

I believe that, for some of us, social media and smartphone use has the potential to tip from habit to addiction. Addiction is a spectrum issue – not everyone who drinks or tries drugs becomes addicted, and not everyone on social media is addicted, but likely some are. It depends. I absolutely don't believe that it's universal and that we are *all* addicted to our phones, and I don't think it's helpful for us to talk about it as if it affects all of us. But neither do I think we should be minimising the potential influence social media can have over us, whether it's our relationships, work, politics or health. What particularly interests me is the influence social media has over our food choices, and how this impacts on our overall wellbeing.

Food pics or it didn't happen

I once overheard someone in a restaurant say: "The calories just aren't worth it if I can't take a good photo for Instagram." That's depressing. Food is one of the most popular things to post about online. Searching for posts using #food on Instagram yields over 350 million results, which isn't all that surprising.* We eat with our eyes; merely seeing beautiful pictures of food can make us salivate, start cravings, or bring forth memories of that food. Research shows that posting photos of food can also be satisfying and beneficial. Taking a quick snap of our food delays the act of eating it, which builds anticipation and contributes to us enjoying the wonderful flavours of that food more. We are now taking so many pictures of our food that manufacturers have released cameras with a specific food mode, and are marketing lenses as being ideal for food photography.

* This is just in English, the most commonly used language on Instagram. If you add the translation of #food into other languages on top of this then the figures are even higher.

Perhaps it's no wonder, then, that 63% of 13–32-year-olds have posted on social media a photo of food or drinks either they, or someone else, were having, and 57% have posted about what they're eating. More people have posted their food than a photo of new clothes they've recently purchased and 19% of young people have even borrowed someone else's food to take a picture of it for Instagram, presumably because it's more attractive.

Pizza is the most popular Instagrammed food worldwide, with sushi and chicken taking second and third place respectively, although in the UK it's curry in the top slot. No surprises there. At the time of writing, the most liked picture on Instagram is one of an egg. Just a single egg on a white background. Someone created an account with the deliberate goal of dethroning Kylie Jenner as having the most popular Instagram photo ever, and they succeeded. What a time to be alive.

Away from Instagram, the 'food and drink' category on Pinterest is the second most popular category, just behind arts and crafts. Among active and regular users of the platform, around half say that Pinterest is their go-to source of food inspiration, while 84% of daily pinners stated they try something new that they have seen on Pinterest at least once a week.

But why is this? Why are we so eager to take and share pictures of food? Actually, there are a number of reasons:

- Because making something ourselves is a source of pride.
- Because we want to record an event or social occasion, or because it's a special treat we want to remember.
- Because the food is beautiful, unusual or different.
- Because we want to track what we're eating – apparently 23%

of all Instagram users photograph their food for a photo-blog or as a food diary.

- Because it says something about ourselves that we want to amplify.

There are few things that can bring people closer together the same way that sharing a meal does. Even if that sharing experience happens via the tap of a button on a screen rather than across a table, there's something special about food. We especially love sharing food online, because it means we don't have to physically give our food away.

Food porn

Food porn videos are the third most viewed video content on the Internet, after music videos and actual porn. Food porn is typically used on platforms such as Facebook or Instagram, captioning delicious and visually appealing food items just before they're about to be eaten. The term 'food porn' goes back to 1979, when Michael Jacobson, co-creator of the Center for Science in the Public Interest in Washington, DC, wanted to contrast healthy and unhealthy foods. He termed the healthy foods 'Right Stuff', and the unhealthy ones 'Food Porn'. Jacobson later clarified that he "coined the term to connote a food that was so sensationally out of bounds of what a food should be that it deserved to be considered pornographic".

Isn't it funny how 'food porn' has gone from being something obscene and awful to something desirable? It's a fetishisation of food. Many young consumers share pictures of the food they eat online and 47% now say they consider themselves foodies. It's no wonder the #foodporn trend has exploded. On Instagram alone there are currently well over 200 million public pictures tagged as food porn.

Choosing or making food that is Instagrammable is an increasingly key part of the decision-making process for millennials, so the time for foods with vibrant colours has arrived. While Instagram-friendly food can be more or less nutritious, ranging from pure fruit smoothie bowls to giant pizzas, food porn is notable for being high calorie and high fat – a direct backlash against diet food. An examination of 10 million Instagram posts tagged with #foodporn found that sugary desserts, particularly chocolate, dominated over all other foods across most of the 72 countries in Instagram's database. Sweet foods seem to be the ultimate food porn.

Of course social media is the place where food porn thrives. The very nature of food porn is that it is consumed visually rather than orally. This also explains why food porn in general is linked more to food eaten out of home rather than to homemade food. Since the term first appeared, food porn has typically referred to watching others cook on television or ordering something in a destination restaurant, rather than cooking something at home. As with regular porn, we enjoy watching what we ourselves presumably cannot do or have. The food becomes a performative piece where flavour is no longer the primary purpose. Food where taste isn't the priority?! Before the advent of mainstream media this would have been almost unthinkable, and yet now it's incredibly common.

Thanks to social media food porn, eating is no longer just an activity. It's an aesthetic.

This visual, performative nature of food is having an impact on the food and restaurant industries. The foods that go viral on social media are not necessarily the ones that taste best but the ones that look best. Arguably, an effective marketing strategy would therefore be first to have a solid social media presence, and second to make food that goes viral. Taste doesn't go viral, looks do.

When Instagram-friendly foods go viral, they can completely change what we choose to eat. One of the greatest examples is avocado toast. Breakfast used to be a chore, something that we had to do in the morning to get on with our day. Now, rather than charred toast with jam or a bowl of soggy cereal, we have the bright photogenic colours of green avocado on toast with juicy red tomatoes. As a result, avocado toast has become a staple in every cafe in major cities like London, New York and Sydney.

You won't find a lot of old-fashioned foods on Instagram, as #food and #foodporn look more to the future than the past – partly because platforms like Instagram are populated with millennials. Instead, you'll find foods that are colourful, exciting and over-the-top, like freakshakes* or 30-inch pizzas.

Social media has meant, more often than not, that we are eating with our eyes as opposed to our other senses. This has placed pressure on restaurants and cafes to up their game and produce ever increasingly photogenic food. If it's not Instagram-worthy, then is it even worth serving?

When these beautiful foods are shared and go viral, the

---

* Freakshakes are milkshakes piled with vast quantities of toppings, including cream, cake, sauce, sweets and any other desired indulgences. They are enormous and striking, designed to be photographed before eating.

restaurants or locations that sell them become go-to destinations, to the point where the food sells out every week, or there are queues out the door, often simply because of one item on the menu. Everyone wants a piece of it, and we suffer from serious FOMO, feeling left out when our feed is full of these items that we haven't tried yet. Once we have, though, it strengthens that community tie on social media and makes us feel good about ourselves that we're in on the action.

We've always eaten with our eyes first, and social media's #foodporn is an amplification of this. It's exciting, it's taking a bit of extra care when plating up a dish, or it's prolonging that anticipation when you've finally ordered a menu item that all your online friends are raving about. It adds to the whole experience of eating.

Food is a social thing

Eating has, throughout history, been seen as a social activity, which is why understanding the social context of food is integral when trying to identify eating patterns. Social media is one of the most significant social revolutions to happen in the world of food and health. Therefore in order to understand why food is one of the most popular subjects online, we need to understand food as a social thing.

Our very first experience of food and eating is a social one: it's a shared experience between parent and child. Food is the most important thing a mother gives her newborn child; it is the substance of her own body and is a symbol of both love and safety. Making and sharing food is, in most cultures, a gesture of love. We give someone cupcakes to show we care about them, chocolates to say sorry, a cake to offer congratulations, or a heart-shaped pizza to express love.

We have to eat in order to live, but food is so much more than simply the nutrients and energy we need to sustain life. The way we cook our food is unique to humans and sets us apart from other animals, but the way we eat together is an animal drive. And because we eat together, food becomes a symbol of our social standing as well as our cultural connections.

In the words of two academics, David Bell and Gill Valentine, "The history of any nation's diet is the history of the nation itself, with food fashion, fads and fancies mapping episodes of colonialism and migration, trade and exploration, cultural exchange and boundary making." A culture is often defined by the foods its people consume. If I say 'France' you think cheese, baguettes and wine. If I say 'India' you think curry and spice. Germany? Beer and sausages. Thailand? Pad Thai. Vietnam? Pho. Morocco? Tagine.

Take a moment to think of one occasion, celebration or holiday that does not involve food in some fundamental way. I can't think of one. Many of our interactions with people we care about involve food and eating, or at the very least drinking tea or coffee. Aside from the social atmosphere surrounding food intake, there exists a powerful dynamic between the social situation and sharing food, including the social norms that govern eating. In many cultures, the importance of food and eating extends well beyond simply providing fuel – it also plays a role in identity expression, communication, celebration, understanding social status and gender roles. The social meaning of food can affect what, how and why we eat.

Now we have more ways of using food as a social tool than ever before. Food blogs, food forums and food groups on social networks are plentiful. Some mostly function as a means to share recipes or food diaries, while others are for reviewing restaurants or dining experiences.

Even when statistics indicate that we eat alone more than half the time, food always connects us to others in some way, whether it's the people who prepare our food, those who grow or harvest it, the other groups of people who eat the same things we do, or the people we share our food with online. When we share food on social media, we deliberately invite other people to participate in our eating experience. By posting about our food on social media, we never truly eat alone. Apparently, the best time for a restaurant to post on Instagram is when people are eating while scrolling through images on their phones: at 9 a.m., between noon and 1 p.m., and around 7–8 p.m.

Food is culture, celebration, comfort, power and identity. In conveying who we are to other people, we use our bodies to project information about ourselves. This is done through the way we move, the clothes we wear, the way we speak, our facial expressions, and the food we consume. Food choices tell us about a person's beliefs, passions, background, knowledge, assumptions and personality.

Research back in the 1980s showed how strong the link is between the foods we eat and how we are perceived by others. People who eat fast food were seen as more religious and likely to be wearing polyester clothing, health foodies were perceived as more left-wing, vegetarians were seen as pacifists who drive foreign cars, and gourmet diners were seen as liberal, sophisticated individuals. The research may be decades old, but diet-based stereotypes are definitely still alive and well. We are much more likely to assume someone who does yoga is also vegan, that a weightlifter eats a meat-heavy high-protein diet, or that someone who has a Sunday roast every week is a traditionalist who likes routine and control. We've seen media headlines that take this to the extreme, stating that if you enjoy bitter foods like gin you're probably a sociopath (you're not, don't worry), and that people who like spicy foods are adrenaline junkies and risk takers (or, in their culture, spice might just be the norm?), and while these are taken a little too far, the basic principle still stands: we make assumptions about people based on their food choices.

To give a more recent example of this: researchers asked university students to rate individuals based on their diets. They were presented with two profiles, who were deliberately chosen because they looked incredibly similar. One of these two profiles was classified as the 'good' eater who ate 'good' foods, and the other was classified as the 'bad' eater. When asked their opinions on these individuals, the students rated the 'good' eater as being more active, attractive, likeable, practical and analytical, as well as thinner than the 'bad' eater. All this despite the fact the profiles were almost identical. Essentially, when we perceive someone as eating 'good' foods (whatever that means both on a societal level and to us personally) we attach other positive and desirable character attributes to them.

Other studies reported a more varied picture when participants read a description of a woman who ordered either a 'good' lunch (chicken sandwich and salad) or a 'bad' lunch (hamburger and fries). Although the eater of the 'good' lunch was seen as having greater moral integrity, people stated they would rather hang out and be friends with the eater of the 'bad' lunch. People who eat 'junk' food and takeaways are perceived as less attractive, less intelligent and less warm, but are also seen as more fun to be around and more likely to go to parties where they will drink alcohol.

Overall, we see people who eat 'good' and 'healthy' food as 'good' people, but also as goodie-two-shoes. People who eat 'bad' and 'unhealthy' foods, on the other hand, are the 'bad guys' who get into trouble but make life interesting.

There is also a clear gender divide in the way we judge people for their food choices. Our assumptions about men aren't really affected by how much they eat, whereas women definitely are judged. We rate women as being more physically attractive when the description of them mentions they eat smaller meals. The catch: this only applies when we can't see the woman, so we're just going on words or visuals of the food. When we can see the woman in front of us, we tend to judge based on her physical appearance or the type of food she's eating, not how much. This makes sense when you consider that, without a visual cue of her body, we fill in the blanks in our minds with the cues around us, such as the amount of food eaten. This especially applies to social media accounts that purely focus on images of food without any real consistent indicator of what the person behind it looks like. We take those food images and make assumptions about the creator's appearance.

In addition to physical attractiveness, it has also been consistently shown that people perceive those who eat smaller meals as being neater, and those who eat larger meals as messier and sloppier. This is likely because Western society equates eating less with discipline, willpower and self-control.

The current emphasis on dieting and slimness in so many

cultures comes packaged with certain norms dictating what and when we should eat, in order to reach a certain body shape and size that is deemed acceptable and desirable. Taken together, these considerations suggest that what we eat has important implications for social judgements. Understanding the social dynamics of food and eating can help us to better understand the social forces that influence people's eating behaviour, including in online social situations – that is, social media.

These assumptions and stereotypes can be manipulated to achieve a particular outcome. For example, Western politicians use this to appeal to the 'everyday working man' by eating everyday foods like burgers, hotdogs, bacon sandwiches and local delicacies to demonstrate that they are part of the community. This has given us some hilariously awful images over the years of politicians either struggling to maintain some dignity or revealing just how out of touch they are by eating a hotdog with a knife and fork.*

What we eat gives the world an image of us; it immediately tells people a number of things about who we are. Is it any wonder that we now spend so much time telling the world what we eat via social media?

Taking a food photo before uploading it to the various social media platforms serves several purposes. It shows we appreciate

---

* There are endless entertaining images and examples online, including: Donald Trump eating KFC with cutlery on a private plane, Hillary Clinton brandishing a pork chop like a weapon, and David Cameron eating a hotdog with a knife and fork. Ed Miliband's infamous battle with a bacon sandwich was thought to have lost him the general election in the UK, as his awkwardness came to signify to his opponents that he wouldn't be able to handle running the country.

our food and have a sense of pride over it, but it is also a way for us to project a particular image of ourselves to others, so they perceive us how we want them to. Our broadcasted images of what we eat help to reflect and express our individuality and lifestyle choices.

Consuming identity

Some of you may remember an online virtual reality game called *Second Life*. In this game, the users, who are called 'residents', design an avatar for themselves and then live any kind of life they desire in the online world through their avatar. Unlike similar games such as *World of Warcraft*, there are no quests, no specific objectives other than creating their dream life. Users can travel around the online world, participate in events such as concerts, lectures or fashion shows, work their dream job, and they can meet other residents and chat to them. Research into this online world has found that, despite the participants' ability to create and perform any kind of identity on *Second Life*, people tended to recreate their offline selves online. Rather than come up with an entirely new fantasy identity, they would start by modelling their current identity, and then simply add their dreams onto it.

While on holiday in Sicily, on an excursion up Mount Etna, I encountered a couple who met on *Second Life*. I was told it was "a bit of an embarrassing story", but convinced them to share. He lived in the Netherlands, she lived in Canada; he had just gone through a divorce while she was still unhappily married. They met online, started falling for each other, and then, once she had begun her divorce proceedings, she flew over to spend two weeks with him. At the end of their time together, when she was crying on the plane back home, she knew that he was the man for her, and ended up moving all the way to Europe to be with him. When she told me this story in 2019, they had been together for twenty years, and married for ten of those. If they had been presenting an identity online that was too far removed from reality, I don't believe they would have fallen in love, as the discrepancy would have felt like a lie. They agreed with this, reaffirming the idea that they were simply being a slightly better version of themselves online.

A lot of influencers on social media are now hosting events and meeting their followers in real life. When I have met some of them, they have been surprisingly different from how they present online (usually in the sense that they are much happier and kid-friendly online), but others have been pretty much exactly the same. Our virtual identities are often just an extension or slight exaggeration of parts of ourselves, the parts we want to magnify. Is this lying? I used to think so, but now I'm not so sure. I don't think this is all that different from how we amplify part of ourselves at work to create a better impression, or try and show our most fun selves on a first date. Is putting on a business suit for work really that different from adding a filter to your photo?

Social media has made our private lives public. This erosion between private and public has spread beyond those who are famous and those who wish to be famous. Every day, ordinary people post their words and images online for all the world to see. The rise of the online microcelebrity and super-public presence has led to a social condition that has been dubbed 'strange familiarity'. This term originates from the sociologist Stanley Milgram who used the term 'familiar strangers' to refer to those people we know based on sight but not by name. This could be someone who is always on the same commuter train with us, someone who lives across the street, or someone we regularly see at the same spin class. While we wouldn't engage in conversation with each other (especially on the Tube – the horror!) we may simply acknowledge each other's existence with a quick nod, or simply a glance of recognition. This applies to familiar strangers we meet in the real world, but how does this apply when we find ourselves sitting in the same cafe as someone whose videos we watch every week as soon as they're uploaded? Or someone we follow on Instagram? Do we engage? How do we navigate this 'strange familiarity'? Many of us react in the same way we would if we saw a celebrity – take a sneaky picture without them noticing and send it to our friends to enjoy and discuss together. An acknowledgement without engagement.

Identity now belongs to the consumer of content, not the creator. Other people who view your content and, by extension, your identity in a public online space will feel a sense of ownership over who you are. They believe that through watching you online they know you in some way. When you behave in a way that matches their assessment of you they are happy and engage with what you have to say, and when you behave in a way they didn't expect, they can feel hurt and betrayed, despite never having met you. This can lead to people becoming incredibly hostile when they feel you've changed in a way they don't agree with, and can contribute to online public shaming and trolling.

Why is everyone better than me?

Of course, the online world of food isn't all sunshine and rainbows. Sharing pictures of your food invites assumptions, judgements and shaming. And following food accounts invites food comparison.

On the surface, our obsession with social media and the validation it offers seem pretty harmless. Even though receiving likes on social media triggers the dopamine system, it is misleading to compare looking at your phone to snorting a line of cocaine. The two are not the same. However, there's no denying that the further we go down the rabbit hole of how social media is affecting our health, the more there seems to be cause for concern.

We know social media can have a significant negative impact on our wellbeing. Spending large amounts of time on social media can increase someone's risk of depression, anxiety, or developing body image issues, eating disorders and low self-esteem. What explains this link between social media and mental health is social comparison.

Humans are thought to possess a fundamental drive to compare themselves with others, which serves a variety of functions, such as a sense of belonging, self-evaluation and reflection, decision-making, inspiration, and regulating emotions and wellbeing. Upward social comparison occurs when we compare ourselves to those who are similar but slightly better than us at something, whereas downward social comparison occurs when we compare ourselves to those who are slightly worse. Although upward social comparison can be beneficial when it inspires people to become more like their comparison targets, and encourages them to do better, more often than not it causes individuals to feel inadequate.

Historically, social comparisons in offline contexts revolved around in-person interactions with people close to us, such as friends, family and co-workers; meaning our comparisons would be limited to a small number of people. But now our increasing use of social media is exposing us to large numbers of people, often strangers, who we establish some kind of connection with, and who we can therefore engage in upward social comparison with. This is because social media platforms allow for carefully curated self-presentation. We have huge amounts of control over what information we share: we decide what content appears on our profiles, we post the pictures we want, and we write posts that describe only the parts of our experiences we choose to. We present our ideal selves online, our best bits, our highlight reel, and everyone else is doing the same. When we then compare our everyday offline lives to the highlight reel we see online (usually from others, although we can compare our online and offline selves) we make an upward social comparison and we fall short. We feel worse about ourselves, as if we're not good enough, and as if our lives aren't exciting and perfect enough.

The figures confirm this: 88% of people engage in making social comparisons on social media, and 98% of these are upward social comparisons. That's a lot of potential opportunities for us to feel dissatisfied with ourselves. In fact, frequent Facebook users believe that the people on their friends list are happier and more successful in life than they are, especially when comparing themselves to people they don't know well offline, or have lost touch with.

Social media also offers up information that isn't typically conveyed easily and explicitly in offline social comparison situations, because our online profiles contain information about our social network. This includes information such as the number of friends or followers and how much engagement someone has with the members of that network. For example, someone who receives plenty of likes and comments on their posts may be an upward comparison target in terms of their popularity or perceived social capital. So online we can see both 'personal' comparison information, such as career success and attractiveness, and 'social' comparison information about their friendships, connections and popularity.

We use this comparison with others to determine what and how much to eat, how we feel about our own food, how we feel about ourselves, and how we feel about others who eat similarly to or differently from us. All this comparison can, understandably, lead to some more serious concerns such as body dissatisfaction, eating disorders, depression and anxiety.

A democratisation of food and health?

Social media is so full of misinformation, yet many people are turning to social media to seek out health information and trust it too.

A survey by the Pew Research Center showed that a shocking 90% of Americans aged 18-24 years have indicated they would trust medical information found on social media, while 42% of American adults would read health information they find on social media and consider changing their behaviours as a result.

Another survey, The Great American Search for Healthcare Information, found that most Americans who regularly seek health information online are concerned that what they are reading is incorrect or misleading, and few have found health information on social media to be accurate. This was consistent across generations.

This is an issue because the democracy of social media means anyone can create a platform and start spouting shit. And so many do. As few as 1% of all healthcare professionals use social media to carry out science communication work through publishing blogs, writing tweets or creating images for Instagram that are aimed at the general public. Which means that everyone else out there talking about food and health isn't qualified to give out advice. The balance is very much in favour of unqualified advice.

An article examining alternative cancer cures on the Internet found the quality of information given "had the potential to harm cancer patients if the advice provided was followed". Some of the information about cancer online even goes so far as to actively discourage patients from pursuing effective conventional treatments such as chemotherapy. This is serious, considering those who deviate from conventional cancer treatment are 2.5 times more likely to die within five years.

When researchers looked at the accuracy of information about coeliac disease, 66% of the websites scored less than 50% for accuracy. This was often because of either incomplete information or blatant inaccuracies in the information that was presented. Misleading information about coeliac disease can lead to someone eating a food that makes them feel incredibly unwell, or can lead to unnecessary fear and restriction of foods that are perfectly safe.

As humans we are far more drawn to stories than we are to

numbers. Anecdotes are more appealing and memorable than statistics. Personal stories about food and health are very common on social media, and while they are absolutely valid for that person, they are often not applicable to others. In many cases, in fact, it could be harmful for others to adopt that information for themselves. It can also drive people to more and more extreme ideas and behaviours concerning food.

Brands and restaurants are collaborating with influencers on social media, giving them free meals and products in exchange for promotion and exposure. Food companies are limited in what they can legally claim about a product on their packaging and in their marketing tools, but using influencers can be a sneaky way of getting around that, leading to the spread of yet more misinformation.

What this book aims to do

Social media platforms like Twitter and Instagram haven't been around for long but are already having far-reaching impacts on our health and wellbeing. We are only just starting to appreciate the influence these platforms have over our decisions relating to food and health, both positive and negative, with many of these processes happening without our even being fully aware of them.

Well, maybe we should be aware. This book will guide you through the various ways social media has affected our food choices, our food and restaurant industries, and our food policy. By the end, you'll be armed with the knowledge and tactics to take back control and make social media work in a healthier way for you.

1

THE 'WHAT' AND 'WHO': WHAT'S NORMAL? WHO DO I WANT TO BE LIKE?

Picture a heterosexual couple out for dinner on their first date. They're both a little nervous, understandably so. The woman will likely eat slightly less to appear more feminine, whereas the man will likely eat more in order to appear more masculine. She is more likely to choose something 'light' like a pasta dish (not a salad, because that would be 'boring'), and he is more likely to choose something meaty like a burger or steak, again to reaffirm how manly he is. Interestingly, neither of them will be fully aware they are doing this, but automatically gravitate towards those choices. Both of them are being influenced by societal expectations, as well as by each other.

What this illustrates is that social norms influence our food choices. Social norms have been described as comprising among the least visible, yet most powerful, forms of social control over human behaviour. These norms can occur whether we're sitting across a table from someone in a restaurant or alone. Our food choices are constantly shaped by those around us, physically and virtually, as well as by society, our self-perception, and by expectations. From infancy, we model people's behaviours to learn and to affiliate with others as well as to be liked and socially embedded due to our need to belong.

Eating is generally a social activity in humans. When we're with a group of friends, and they all order a burger, there's a much higher chance that we'll order a burger as well, so that we fit in, even if it's not exactly what we want. No one wants to be the odd one out. The reverse is also true: if we're the only person in a group who's ravenously hungry, chances are we'll eat less to match everyone else. This is essentially a form of people-pleasing – of placing the perceived needs, expectations and desires of others above our own. We will adapt our food intake to that of the person we're eating with, and a group eating together will converge on an eating norm, which reduces the variance between individuals. What this means is that, on average, we tend to eat more when we're in the company of others compared to when we're alone, and the bigger the group the more we eat. This is partly due to the fact that group meals tend to take longer, but it's also because eating together is an enjoyable process. Some people might interpret this to mean 'you should eat alone to avoid gaining weight', but I say screw that. Social eating is what makes us human, plus it helps us live long and happy lives. Besides, eating alone doesn't exactly mean we're free of influence either.

Informational eating norms

Obviously, when we're with others we're affected by societal norms, as well as how we wish to be perceived by the person or people around us. But a huge number of people eat at least some meals alone. Well, almost alone. Most of us will eat with our phones right next to us, or while scrolling and reading. Our phones and our access to social media are always there, influencing us between mealtimes as well.

Humans are social creatures, and we have evolved to adapt to the group standard in order to keep that sense of community and belonging. We use the behaviour of others as a guide for how we should behave, and adhere to this even when we believe we are alone and not being watched. When it comes to eating behaviour in particular, we see what others eat and use that to inform our own food decisions. The extent to which we believe others are eating healthily or unhealthily can also influence our choices. If we feel like everyone around us is eating 'healthily' then we're inclined to do the same. This explains why concordance in eating habits is observed in social networks – including online social networks.

A person doesn't have to be sitting opposite you to influence your food choices. Simply having information about other people's eating habits is enough to influence what we eat and how much. This is known as informational social influence. Informational social influence is when we make use of the behaviour of those around us to decide whether a course of action is adaptive (meaning if everyone else is doing it, it will probably be a good idea for me to do it too). Through informational eating norms we discover information about the eating habits of people, which could be communicated through explicit written information or cues about the typical eating behaviour of others. This effect is just as powerful as having someone eating at a table with you.

There are many examples of this in the research, where written information about what food other people had been eating, or what they typically chose, affected people's decisions. This can be in the form of an observation ('pasta is really popular at our work canteen') or from visual cues, such as graphs. When we are given cues that others around us eat large portions of food, we're more likely to eat more, and vice versa. In numerous studies, informational food choice norms have also been shown to have a consistent effect on food choice. Norms can influence our intake of snack food, fruit and vegetables, and main meals.

One of the studies, which I love, focused on chocolate (that's why I love it). The number of chocolates taken by visitors in the lunchroom at work was much higher when there were some empty chocolate wrappers in the bowl, because this indicated that the norm was for everyone (or most people) to take a chocolate. This effect worked even though the visitors never saw anyone else take a chocolate – the wrappers were evidence enough.

This effect is measurable regardless of body size, gender, weight, hunger or age. In other words: everyone does it. The effect tends to be stronger with snack foods than with fruits and vegetables, likely because people tend to be more confident in their likes and dislikes when it comes to these. It's also likely because we tend to be pretty confident that the upper limit for what is deemed a socially acceptable amount of fruit and vegetables is pretty damn high, whereas what is an appropriate quantity of snack foods like cookies or crisps is more up for debate.

Although everyone is affected by norms, we're more likely to respond to a norm if it comes from people we identify with in some way. Let's take an example, where the workers on the day shift at a workplace have a preference for pasta but those on the night shift prefer curry. A new recruit who joins the day shift and learns of both preferences will likely deliberately choose to avoid the curry because it is the preference of the 'other' group. In studies, if participants were told that an undesirable social group really liked this food, and then they were offered as much as they wanted, they would eat far less than usual. This reinforces the idea that conforming to social norms is a way of identifying with a particular group, which is in line with social identity theory. You could therefore make the case that if someone feels a strong sense of community, and that community is perceived to be trying to eat healthily, that person would then also try to eat healthily to maintain a consistent sense of social identity.

Of course, we're also more likely to change our behaviour to match a norm if it's coming from people who we're really close to, like friends and family. Our families are particularly important when it comes to learning food norms when we're younger, and then as we grow up the primary influence gradually shifts more towards friends and colleagues.

Overall, what the research suggests is that some people will have a greater influence over our food choices and intake than others. Women may also be more affected because of greater empathy for others, and because the societal pressures to conform to the thin ideal are much more powerful. Regardless of gender, though, norms will have a stronger impact on you if they are tied more closely to a group that matters to you, such as family, close friends, or even a food community online. The more strongly you identify with a group the more power the norms of that group have over you, and few places have stronger food communities than social media.

In fact, more recently, researchers have started looking at norms and social modelling behaviour on social media and have found that we model the eating of people we interact with on social media. For example, when participants received information that the person who they were interacting with online had eaten more sweets, they themselves ate more as well. When the other person didn't eat anything, participants tended also to match that, and eat no sweets at all, even if they claimed afterwards that they were hungry. Interestingly, those who felt less satisfied with their bodies and had lower self-esteem did this much more strongly than those who were comfortable in themselves.

Often when we start down a path of eating a certain way, we want to surround ourselves (virtually) with people who eat in similar or near-identical ways, especially if we cannot find those people in our immediate friend group. Also, if someone is in the early stages of adopting a way of eating, they might want to test the waters online first before making it a big deal in real life. In this way, social media has its communities of food identities: Slimming World, WW, paleo, vegan, raw vegan, carnivore, flexitarian, macrobiotic, clean eating and so on. These are constantly reinforced through usernames (for example, @jenny_slimmingworld) and hashtags (e.g. #vegan, #keto, #eatclean). If you were suddenly to see everyone in your social media community eating a particular food you'd want to join in too, and be far more likely to buy that food and post about it in order to fit in.

Approval from our peers informs and affects our behavioural intentions. Social media is one of the easiest forms of external validation and ways to gain approval. Simply posting a picture of your food on Instagram or posting a check-in at a popular restaurant on Facebook then allows others to show their approval by liking or commenting on your posts, reinforcing the social norm.

Back in my wellness days, #PancakeSunday was a big trend on Instagram. Over the course of a month it felt like almost everyone I was following was eating pancakes on the same day. I felt left out, I felt like I wasn't in on the trend, so I started making pancakes too, every Sunday, even if I didn't want them. It was purely so I could take a picture for the 'gram and ride that bandwagon. None of my family members or friends were doing this. It had nothing to do with my face-to-face relationships with people, and yet their indifference didn't have anywhere near as much of an impact as those likes, comments and follows I was getting every weekend.

This is the power of social media; it opens you up to new social norms that are outside your immediate circle. Sometimes this is a good thing. Someone from an extremely conservative family can learn about feminism and equality; someone from a small country town can see the LGBT+ trends and norms in big cities, and we can learn about the norms of other cultures. But when it comes to food, the effect seems to be less about gaining inspiration, and more about new communities with strict rules and norms from which you can be virtually cast out at any moment. It's an extra pressure on top of interpersonal social norms.

In particular, what large influencers post on social media about their food can have consequences on you, the followers. We see large numbers of likes and follows and we're more likely to join in, more likely to listen, less likely to question. These influencers have a disproportionate amount of visibility, and as such can shift perceptions of what is 'normal' much more easily.

It doesn't matter if the photo is of someone eating, or the photo is simply of the food. The message is still the same: I'm eating this. Because the image is attached to a profile, to someone whose appearance we are likely aware of, and know to be a real person, it doesn't matter if we actually see them eating it or not, we make that association in our minds. It still has the same influence over our food decisions.

What's trending?

Just like #PancakeSunday, there are endless food trends on social media, ranging from the delicious to the absurd. We've had:

* Moralisation of food, for example 'real' food or 'clean' eating.
* Brightly coloured smoothie bowls (which now mostly consist of just frozen bananas and some other ingredient to give it colour, often blue algae... tasty...).
* Buddha bowls. These are usually vegan, and have a mixture of grains, protein and vegetables artfully arranged side by side in a bowl. Technically, it's not a buddha bowl until you've taken a picture of it and posted it online. Otherwise, it's really just a segmented salad. Oh, and it has nothing to do with Buddha.
* In fact, everything in bowls. Plates are so 2009.
* More extreme eating labels, like raw vegan, fruitarian, keto and carnivore (more on these in chapter 3).
* Macro counting and IIFYM (If It Fits Your Macros).
* Endless powdered substances that allegedly replace fruits and vegetables (they don't).

... and so on.

These trends often grow exponentially. People are much more likely to hit that 'like' button on images that have already received plenty of attention and likes from others, especially their friends. Aside from simple subconscious conformity, there's a sense that we must be missing something if we don't like it too. It's a real sense of FOMO and worry. Did we not get the joke? Are we unaware of a new trend? Is this something we're supposed to think is cool?

One example of a big trend that owes a lot to social media is veganism, by which I mean that its rise in popularity is largely down to the Internet. Even though there are far more vegetarians in the world than vegans, Google searches and Instagram hashtags are higher for #vegan than #vegetarian.

Veganism has been linked to key movements over the last few years: compassion and inclusivity, sustainability, and health. It is also subject to much more controversy than vegetarianism, which drives more headlines and articles on the subject. But what has had arguably the biggest effect on the rise of veganism has been the fact that it's been driven by millennials, and millennials are the first social media generation. While we may not have grown up with social media from birth, we were the first generation to adopt platforms like Facebook and Instagram in large numbers. Millennials and Gen Z spend far more time on social media than our baby-boomer counterparts.

So any movement popular among young people is going to feature heavily on social media, and veganism is no exception. The vegan community are incredibly active on social media. Their choices are driven by strong fundamental beliefs and a passion that's evangelical in nature. Social media is the ideal platform to share such ideas – anyone can create an account and start posting. YouTube and Instagram in particular are full of influencers answering every question imaginable about veganism, showing what they eat in a day, and debunking common myths and misconceptions.

In the past, a movement might have needed mainstream media coverage to be able to share its message. But social media lets users find information naturally rather than having it forced on them. Someone might not deliberately seek out information on veganism, but come across it simply by scrolling through their social media feed and start reading. This helps the movement grow organically. Social media also allows people to find inspiration. Veganism still isn't that common, and while someone might not have any friends or family who eat the same way, they can find happy and thriving influencers online who have already pre-empted their questions and created content-providing answers. Some of this content works specifically to dispel potential myths. For example, there's still a common belief that vegans struggle to obtain enough protein from plants, and that can be easily corrected online. Veganism as a movement tends to favour young people, the very same people who are most likely to be on social media and to seek information on social media.

Online there's a clear and understandable desire to prove that veganism is fun and delicious, not restrictive. Of course, it can absolutely be too restrictive for some and there is still a misconception that vegan food is 'rabbit food' – bland and tasteless. This desire to prove that vegan food is exciting and tasty lends itself especially well to visual platforms like Instagram, Pinterest and YouTube. In fact, a 2018 article in the *Independent* directly linked the rise of Instagram with the growth of veganism. Instagram is a creative platform, and making vegan versions of popular foods taste good does require some creativity, something which vegan cooks often display in abundance.

While I think it's admirable that veganism is growing, I also think it's important to say that it's not for everyone, and it shouldn't be made out to be a simple choice. Not long ago I had the chance to facilitate a panel discussion with Gen Z individuals on their views of veganism. Most of them stated they feel pressured to go vegan, and that this pressure comes from a number of sources, including social media. By all means go vegan if you want to, but not because you feel your friends will judge you for not doing so, or because it'll get you more likes on Instagram, or because you think it's the only acceptable way to eat. It's not.

Who do you want to compare yourself to?

Eating behaviours are hugely affected by social norms, but can also be viewed through the lens of comparison. Historically, social comparison was considered to be the outcome of a basic and ubiquitous human drive to evaluate how correct our opinions are and how good our abilities are in the context of the people around us. However, this understanding was soon expanded to include our evaluation of other qualities and behaviours, such as our emotions.

As a reminder, when we compare ourselves to better-off or superior others this is upward social comparison. When we compare ourselves to worse-off or inferior others this is downward social comparison. These social comparisons can occur in the context of a number of behaviours: intelligence, grades, sports, finances and, of course, eating behaviours. For example, children will very quickly complain that a sibling received a bigger portion of a favourite food than they did. In such cases, the effect of the comparison might affect how the child feels and might also influence the child's eating behaviour at the next meal. For example, they might eat more of something else because they feel they deserve to compensate for missing out earlier. But, of course, adults engage in this comparison too, even though we like to think we don't. Many people will adamantly insist they don't engage in comparison, but the important thing to note is that this is largely an automatic, unconscious process.

We are far more likely to compare our plates of food to another person's if they are perceived to be similar to us in some way. As a 27-year-old woman I am not really going to compare my food to a 60-something-year-old man, but I would absolutely compare with my female flatmate who is just two years older than me.

Most people tend to look at each other while eating together, that much is obvious, and while we may be mainly focused on our own plate, we are taking note of everyone else's as well. Even if we're eating alone, we're comparing our food to the people we follow on social media, and evaluating our choices based on that information. When we're being watched while we eat, we feel self-conscious and eat less, as if we feel our eating becomes excessive when compared with the person watching who isn't eating at all. Not that this is a common real-life scenario, but even the thought of it does feel a little uncomfortable.

To illustrate how this comparison affects our eating habits, I want to share a recent study about pizza. Participants were given a standard slice of pizza, and were told this was a 'light lunch' before a taste perception study in which they would share their opinions with another (actually non-existent) participant. Under this false premise, the real purpose of the study was to see how the participants responded to comparing the size of their pizza slices. Although all participants were given a slice of pizza of the same size, a third of them saw a smaller slice pass by them to be given to the fictitious other participant, another third saw a larger slice going past, and the remaining third were given no comparison opportunity. So, although all the participants received an identical slice of pizza, two-thirds of them were able to compare it to the fake participant's slice size. Because of this comparison, a third thought they had been given a large piece and a third thought they had been given a small piece. Those participants who were on a diet were disappointed if they had been given a smaller piece, as they thought they had missed out on an opportunity to (be required to) eat more of a delicious, often 'forbidden' food.

In a subsequent study with the same design, when participants were then offered more pizza afterwards, those who thought they had received a smaller slice compensated by eating more pizza than those who thought they had received a larger slice. So, really, we're just like children in that regard, worrying that we're missing out.

Comparing our food to others also affects how much we like our own meal, which in turn affects how much of it we eat. Studies have shown that, if I were to give you a sandwich when you know your friend is getting a pizza, your (understandable) disappointment will mean you eat less of the sandwich and don't enjoy it as much. But if you're the one with the pizza while your friend longingly looks on, soggy sandwich in hand, you're likely to eat more pizza and enjoy it more too. Schadenfreude really is a thing!

It's important to add that people on a diet tend to be especially influenced by comparison with what others are eating. Dieters are more likely to be more concerned about what they and others around them are eating, and more likely to use others as a guide. On the other hand, individuals with total food freedom who are more body confident are less likely to be concerned that others perceive them as eating 'too much' compared to others, or eating 'bad' foods that aren't permitted on their diet.

We're all more likely to engage in social comparison in unfamiliar situations or when we feel uncertain. For example, eating at a dinner table with a group of strangers may promote more comparison than eating at a table with close friends. If those strangers are people you want to impress, the stakes are even higher and the chance of comparison even greater. The first time you eat in a country you haven't visited before you'll likely search around you for clues on what's acceptable to eat and model the behaviour of others in terms of how to eat as well. On a first date your food choices can very much be affected by what and how much the other person is eating (which is why, personally, I don't understand why people go for dinner on a first date, just do drinks!).

We all engage in some form of social comparison in our day-to-day lives. It's part of the unconscious processing going on inside our brains that helps us evaluate who we are in relation to others – an incredibly adaptive survival mechanism. But some of us compare more than others, and some are more affected by it than others. Those people are said to be high in social comparison orientation (SCO). If you're interested, you can find out where you sit on that scale by doing the assessment in the final chapter (see pages 289). In general, individuals who have low self-esteem, seek validation from others more than from within, are perfectionists, are unsure of who they are, are dissatisfied with their bodies, and have low self-confidence tend to engage in more comparison than those who are more secure in themselves. This makes a lot of sense, because people with high self-esteem are more likely to believe that others like them, compared to people with low self-esteem. Those with high self-esteem don't worry as much about how they are perceived by others, and assume rejection by others is less likely, therefore they don't feel the same strong need to affirm social bonds with others. Essentially, the more comfortable you are in your own skin, the less you tend to compare, because you just don't care that much about what others think.

Those high in SCO are incredibly sensitive and aware of others, are less secure, and more uncertain about their self-concept – a collection of the beliefs we hold about ourselves. They are less comfortable in who they are and more likely to take cues from others around them, in order to try and fit in as much as possible. Individuals low in SCO, on the other hand, adopt more of an attitude of 'if they don't like who I am, that's not my problem'.

When comparison has considerable power over us, to the point that it makes us unhappy and feel out of control, that's when it is a problem, and social media is a huge comparison enabler. It offers an ideal platform for comparison to take place. We know we're an incredibly nosy bunch – most social media activity consists of scrolling through others' profiles and content without actually making contact (for example, liking or commenting on something).

Research shows that high SCO individuals tend to use social media more heavily than low SCO individuals. They tend to spend more time online and are more invested. On top of that, they're also more likely to feel worse about themselves after engaging in this online comparison. You'd be forgiven for thinking this doesn't make sense – why would the people who are most likely to experience negative consequences of online comparisons be the ones who spend the most time on it? First, social media is a rich source of comparison material and may therefore appeal, despite the negative consequences. If you're uncertain about yourself, any information about others may feel better than none. Second, people may be claiming to engage in comparison for the purpose of self-improvement, and looking at aspirational content can provide motivation for that. Third, the negative consequences of this online comparison are sneaky and implicit, and we can't necessarily easily connect them to our social media use, as it's likely related to a pattern of behaviour rather than one-off scenarios. This makes it considerably harder to detect and therefore doesn't discourage scrolling and scrolling.

Are you inspired or are you just copying someone?

One of the most obvious and (in my view) problematic ways in which we're able to compare our eating habits to those online is through 'what I eat in a day' content.

Tally Rye is a fitness blogger who used to post what I eat in a day (WIEIAD) videos on a regular basis. "Firstly, I did it because it's what everyone else was doing, because it was easy content, and because it got views. Did I feel the pressure to eat certain things when I was making the videos? Yes. There was more of a thought process behind what I was eating and having to remind myself to grab my camera when I just wanted to grab a snack from the fridge."

Was it an accurate portrayal of her food choices? "It would be around 80% close to what I would eat in a day, but it would be the best version of what I eat in a day. I wanted it to look like everyone else's [videos] and I would focus on the healthy food I ate because that was my brand. Like with any social media posts it was a highlight reel rather than a true reality. I naively assumed that what everyone else was posting in these videos was actually how they ate, and I wanted to be a part of that."

It's important to point out that these videos were coming from a place of simply following norms, and creating something Tally thought was useful for people, based on the feedback she would get. "For a while I thought my WIEIAD videos were helpful to people, but then I read an article [written by a dietitian, which stated the harm they can cause] and I realised it wasn't helpful or necessary for me to post, even though they were my most popular videos. I think people consuming them still feel like they need to be told what to eat and don't trust themselves, and I want people to trust themselves, so I don't think it's right that I share these things."

People who are in the fitness space still post these videos regularly, and I was curious to hear why Tally thought that was the case. She identifies two reasons. "I think [some people still post these videos] because they haven't healed – they're in limbo. Others have never had a bad relationship with food, and they don't see the problem and can't empathise and relate to how others can feel about them." This makes sense to me, as many fitness bloggers come from a background either of eating disorders or performing arts – or both. There is also a pressure to look as fit and healthy as possible, and to show that this came from hard work – from food and exercise – rather than mainly from genetics.

Tally stopped creating these videos and shared her decision in a YouTube video explaining why she had chosen not to post WIEIAD content any longer. Her followers reacted very kindly. By doing this, Tally decided to put her audience's health above her own popularity, which is amazing, but it's also something that most people wouldn't do. Interestingly, she says some other bloggers reacted badly to the video and took it as a personal attack, so she had to have a conversation with them reassuring them that wasn't the case – it wasn't about anyone else, just her view. The very fact that people got so defensive about it does, to me, suggest some level of insecurity.

"A lot of people on social media hate criticism and hate being hated. They're using [these videos] to be liked, and people are scared of not posting them because they want to please people." I agree, there definitely seems to be an element of people-pleasing involved, as well as a need to have your food choices validated and praised by others. Perhaps one or two WIEIAD posters are leaning towards narcissism, but I think it's far more likely that it stems from insecurity and a need to be liked.

I want to outline clearly why I have never and will never share exactly 'what I eat in a day'. What I eat is going to be completely different from one day to the next. It'll depend on how hungry I am, how much time I have, how much I move my body, and whether I go out to eat or cook at home. I'm fully aware of the responsibility I have, both as a healthcare professional and someone who has a large audience on social media. I wouldn't want someone to think that just because I choose to eat something that they should eat it too, or because I don't eat something that it's a 'bad' food that they need to avoid. I'm happy to do a little role-modelling online, but I definitely don't want people to feel guilty for not eating the way I do, or thinking that if they eat like me, they will look like me. Because that's not going to happen. What we eat is so individual that this level of comparison is unhelpful and more likely to harm.

We all have a tendency to get stuck in our food habits, eating the same things every week, buying the same vegetables in our weekly shop. Following food accounts on social media can encourage people to try new ingredients, new cooking methods or whole new cuisines. The images give a great reference point, and it's incredibly accessible. I've seen some great examples of this on Instagram. I've seen food bloggers encourage people to take part in a month-long challenge where they have to try a new vegetable each week, watched eco bloggers show their followers how to make stock from vegetable scraps (seriously, it's incredible!), and I've seen travel food bloggers show people how great it is to get outside your comfort zone and try exciting dishes when travelling abroad.

Social media should be a source of inspiration – that's one of its big benefits. I don't think many of us are going on social media with the intention of engaging in comparison. Sure, we might just be bored, and we're probably opening Facebook for the tenth time that day out of habit, but often we'll tap that icon with the intention of being inspired ("What could I make for dinner?" "What do I do with this fennel?") only to quickly descend into comparison. Inspiration says "I could do that", comparison says "What's the point, it'll never be as good as that." Inspiration says "I want to do better" with curiosity and excitement, whereas comparison says "I'm not as talented as them, I'm not good enough" with jealousy, shame or sadness. Inspiration is motivating, comparison is disheartening.

As Tally acknowledges, "I definitely would follow and look at all these accounts who only posted perfect food, and I wanted to be surrounded by that and felt inspired by that." But did that inspiration tip over into comparison? "Probably... I'm sure it did, and even now I still sometimes have to override these feelings."

I am very much in support of the idea of seeking food inspiration and recipe inspiration online. After all, there are so many wonderful sources out there that have been made far more accessible by the Internet and social media. But there's a big difference between copying a recipe you saw on YouTube that looked delicious and copying someone's entire day of eating.

What do you want people to think of you?

It's important to note that we don't just view food-related content online, we also upload food content to social media platforms. Most of us have, at some point or other, either tweeted about food, posted a 'check-in' on Facebook, or shared a food picture on Instagram. I think it's less interesting that we do this, and more interesting to know *why* we do this.

We've all done those online quizzes: 'Choose your favourite cheese and we'll tell you what career you should have' or 'Pick your favourite carbs to find out what TV show you should watch next' or 'Can we guess your personality based on your favourite takeaway?' They're fun, and they may seem pointless, but there is an element of truth to them: the food we eat tells other people something about us. We use food to portray a certain image or impression to others. This is known as impression management, meaning the processes by which people control how they are perceived by others, often when there is a difference in how they want to be perceived and how they actually are perceived.

The idea of food as a signifier of status is nothing new. Our preference for certain foods has long reflected our social position – for example, being a fan of caviar or lobster. Our food choices themselves therefore become acts of social positioning. What is new, however, is the pace and means by which food is communicated today. Food is no longer seen as simply fuel for the body; it has become currency that can be used online for social status. And one of the ways we can increase our social capital or make ourselves seem cool or popular is by sharing desirable meals and food items through social media. In fact, this is one of the easiest ways we can showcase or increase our status, as we have far more control over our social media pages than we do over our image in real life. We can make more considered, deliberate decisions about what information to put forward for viewing and consumption by others.

In this way, the food we eat and post about it is curated to create a specific image we want to share with the world. While considered and curated, this self-presentation is rarely a deliberate malicious attempt at deceiving others, and more about selectively choosing which parts of ourselves we want to share, and what information to disclose in order to achieve certain social goals or be liked by people who are important to us.

Stereotypes based on eating are interesting in their own right (see the introduction, pages 18–21), but here I want to address an additional element of importance: understanding how these stereotypes may affect our eating behaviour.

First, because eating is usually a social event, it is vulnerable to social influences, including impression management based on consumption stereotypes. In certain situations, we may exploit these stereotypes and eat in a particular way, say eating less than usual, with the intention of projecting a particular aspect of ourselves to others. Second, these stereotypes may be internalised, so they affect how we view ourselves, and can lead to self-criticism. These stereotypes can therefore end up changing our behaviours around food, both in public and in private. We change our behaviours, but we also judge the behaviours of others based on the type and amount of food eaten.

In practice, if we see someone eating foods we deem to be 'good' foods we are more likely to believe that they're a good person. Seems harmless, as we can still have these perceptions corrected by spending more time with that person. But when we internalise these ideas, over time we persuade ourselves that we are a 'bad' person for eating 'bad' foods. Our impression of ourselves becomes distorted, which can drive self-criticism and unhappiness. These ideas take shape over time, with repetition, and can slowly start to take hold of our feelings of self-worth.

In terms of how people respond to these assumptions, stereotypes and impressions, it seems there is both a conscious component whereby we deliberately try to project a socially desirable image to others, and also an unconscious process whereby we may try to maintain this image even when no one is watching. The deliberate aspect is important as we're more likely to make choices based on impression management when we have plenty of time to make a decision, for example when deciding what to post on our social media pages.

Based on the mixed assumptions that are made when someone eats healthily (that they are attractive and smarter but also boring), we may shift our eating habits according to the assumptions we know our audience (either the people we're with or our social media friends/followers) tend to make, so we aim to create a particular impression of ourselves in the eyes of others. If we post a few pictures of 'healthy' food in a row and receive nothing but praise in the comments, then we're likely to continue posting similar images. However, if the response is more along the lines of 'Boring! Don't you ever eat anything fun?' we might choose to post an image of something like a pizza next time to show we can also be fun.

If we wish to be perceived as professional and mature, we might steer clear of posting images of 'childish' foods such as mac and cheese, cookies or other childhood favourites, whereas if we want to be considered both fun and attractive, we might post a picture of ourselves eating a burger – so people can see our face/body for the beauty aspect and the food for the fun bit, thereby combining the two. A fat person who wants to be perceived as healthy and trying to lose weight might only post pictures of healthy meals, partly to portray this impression, but also to avoid being shamed for their food choices online.

Impression management strategies are aimed at disclosing or emphasising the right characteristics. Taken to the extreme, this implies self-marketing and personal branding. I'll admit, I still do this kind of impression management on my social media – to be honest, I think it's unavoidable. I will post pictures of foods like pizza and cookies partly to reassure people that I eat these foods too, that I'm not some 'health freak', and to make myself seem more approachable. People do notice this, although I'm not sure they necessarily consciously connect the dots, because during periods where I haven't posted these kinds of pictures, I've been told I can come across as a kind of 'distant nutrition knowledge machine'. In other words, I'm not as approachable and relatable. Occasionally, I resolve this by not posting any food pictures at all. You could argue that this is my way of creating a personal brand online that is focused on how I want to be perceived by my audience.

We can also be affected by the preferences that are generally displayed in social media communities. We have a tendency to create an echo chamber on social media (particularly on Instagram) whereby we follow people who eat similarly to ourselves, and if a particular kind of food is gaining popularity and positive comments we will be more inclined to buy/cook/order the same thing to give the impression of being popular and part of the group. This can also lead to the food posted on social media being totally unrepresentative of what someone usually eats when alone.

Impression management is particularly of note during times of uncertainty in our lives, for example during adolescence. If impression-management concerns among children and adolescents are more focused on being seen as likeable and fun to be with, rather than being seen as intelligent with moral integrity, then they may choose more 'unhealthy' foods like crisps and chocolate rather than fresh produce like an apple. When teenagers were asked by researchers to note what kinds of foods they associate with someone popular, they pointed out more traditionally 'unhealthy' foods, and particularly branded products, whereas they associated more 'healthy' foods with being unpopular.

All of us now have the ability to create images of ourselves for social purposes without being constrained by time or space. We all have access to the Internet and social media, where we can create strategic profiles and post specific content in the form of images and comments, all to influence how others perceive us.

It's all in the brain

Whether we are aware of the influence that social media has over our food choices or not, it is definitely affecting us. Eating behaviours are determined by eating decisions, which are made in the brain. Our food choices are guided by the visual system, and the sight of food triggers a host of brain responses such as a desire to eat, salivation and preparing to eat, recall of memories from previous times where we've eaten this food, and anticipation of pleasure.

Scientists have observed that when we are shown pictures of food, the amygdala, lateral orbitofrontal cortex and insular cortex in the brain all light up in imaging studies. These areas are all considered part of the appetitive brain network. The amygdala passes information about sensory cues to the lateral orbitofrontal cortex and has an important role in reward processing. The insular cortex receives information about external cues and internal hunger, and it's been suggested its activity relates to memory retrieval of previous experiences with the particular food in the image. What this shows is that the brain's response to images of food is akin to its response to seeing actual food: images stimulate the appetite network in the brain, while also conjuring up memories of previous experiences of that food (or similar foods) to try to remember whether this food is something we've enjoyed in the past. If it is, then it's not surprising that this can make us feel hungry and have a strong desire to eat that food. Such is the powerful influence of just a single food image, let alone an entire feed of them.

A recent study found that young people are aware that food-related posts on social media influence their appetite and their food choices. Researchers found that participants considered social media to be a platform to exchange ideas and information about food. They said that when they see food posts from their friends they feel a desire to have that same food, even if they don't necessarily feel hungry. Of course, sometimes, especially if we're busy and distracted, the sight or thought of food can remind us that we are physiologically hungry. Other times, it's purely a desire for something that looks delicious, without actually feeling hungry. Some participants shared that they have to actively restrain themselves from being influenced by the food pictures on social media.

Overall, it seems that social media can have a significant impact on our food choices. We are influenced by social norms and our desire to fit in, especially when a food is deemed to be trendy. We have a tendency to compare our food to that of others, which can drive us to choose food that we know others will be envious of, and to eat more or less in situations of uncertainty. And we use our food choices as a way to project certain images and perceptions about ourselves, especially in the context of highly curated and selective Instagram posts.

Clearly, social media absolutely influences what we eat in a number of ways. But what about *how* we eat?

2

THE 'HOW': SHOULD I TRACK? BE MINDFUL? PERFORM?

When you think about how social media might have changed *how* we eat, the first thing that tends to come to mind is the antisocial side, the idea that we're using our phones instead of talking to the people we're with. While our phones may allow us to connect with others from almost anywhere at any time, this does come with a downside and a growing concern that our obsession with our phones is distracting us from social interactions. The term 'phubbing' defines the act of snubbing someone in a social setting by concentrating on your phone instead of talking to the person directly and giving them your full attention. There truly is a word for everything.

Most of us would agree that using our phone when we're around others is a bit rude, and yet we keep doing it. As soon as one person in the group starts using their phone, we see that as an open invitation to do the same, and it sends the implicit message that it's socially acceptable to do so. Research shows that the people most likely to be glued to their phone screen while hanging out with friends exhibited lower self-control, greater fear of missing out, and were more likely to show addiction-like behaviours towards their phone.

Yes, we may be whipping our phones out and dividing our attention between social media and our companions, but the far-reaching effects of social media extend beyond that. Through the rise of social media, we've seen a greater interest in food tracking, distracted eating and performative eating.

Should you track what you're eating?

Technology has massively changed *how* we keep track of what we eat as humans. Through tracking apps and devices, we can now meticulously overanalyse every bite we eat, every step we take and every night we sleep. Just like that creepy song by The Police, these trackers are always watching you. Using gadgets to track how much we eat, sleep and exercise is a recent phenomenon, a twenty-first-century obsession.

There's this idea that we need to know every detail about our habits and bodily functions, and that this knowledge is the key to our being healthier and better off. The argument is that information is power, and that therefore it's empowering for us to know all these details about our lives. But while it can seem exciting and insightful, that's not necessarily the case.

Over the past few years, a growing number of articles and personal stories have emerged about how tracking apps, whether for food, sleep or exercise, have fuelled obsessive and unhealthy behaviour. According to sleep researchers, almost half of us are getting less than six hours' sleep each night, and insomnia is on the rise. Many who have struggled with sleep try turning to technology in an attempt to understand their patterns, in the hope that this knowledge will provide answers to improve their sleep. We're now so obsessed with the perfect sleep that researchers have come up with a word for this obsession: ortho-somnia. Did I mention there's a word for everything?

The problem is that for many people, they're actually getting decent sleep, but the app or tracker can register it as disturbed sleep. When they wake up feeling refreshed but the app disagrees, who do they trust? The app, of course. We have a tendency to believe that these trackers must be smarter than what our bodies are telling us, which is absolutely not true. The algorithms used by trackers are complex, for sure, but they are childishly simple in comparison to the processes going on inside our bodies.

Now, you can argue that people know when they've slept badly, and they don't need an app to tell them, but food and movement is different. Dieting and calorie counting obviously aren't new, people have been relying on external guides to tell them what to eat and how to move for decades, but these apps and devices make it so much easier to become preoccupied with numbers.

The science regarding the health benefits of fitness trackers is incredibly underwhelming. Some studies have found a short-term increase in exercise when people first start using their trackers. Long term, however, the benefits often dissipate to the same level as before.

In one randomised controlled trial, working people in Singa-pore were randomly assigned to either an activity tracker, a tracker plus charity incentives, a tracker plus cash incentives, or none of these (the control group). The charity or cash incentives were conditional upon participants achieving a set number of weekly steps, as well as doing some moderate activity. Initially, the cash incentive meant people did, on average, 30 minutes more exercise per week, while the charity incentive led to around 15 minutes extra per week, compared to those without a tracker. However, those effects only lasted a few months. By the time a full year was up, there was no real difference between the four groups of people in terms of activity or health outcomes.

More concerning than the lack of results is the evidence that, for some people, using a fitness tracker can actually result in worse health outcomes. In general, tracking can increase how much movement people do, but it can also turn enjoyable activities into a chore or a job, by focusing too much on the outcome rather than the joy of the process.

Jordan Etkin, Professor of Marketing at Duke University, North Carolina, conducted a number of experiments to examine the effects that tracking had on the amount of each activity that participants completed, and on how much they enjoyed the activities. In the first test, students spent 10 minutes colouring simple shapes. Some were told how many shapes they had coloured as they worked, and those people were more productive than those whose colouring hadn't been tracked. However, the trackers also reported a lower sense of enjoyment, and weren't as creative with their colouring. Their productivity came at the expense of pleasure and creativity.

In the second test, students were asked to record their thoughts for a day while walking. One group was offered the option to wear a pedometer for the day, and almost all of them agreed to wear it. This group were told to regularly keep an eye on the number of steps they had taken. The other group was given a pedometer with the display cover taped shut and told they were wearing it only to test how comfortable it was, so while the researchers could record the number of steps, they themselves didn't know. The group that tracked their own steps walked further, but reported that they enjoyed it less, despite the fact that they had chosen to wear the pedometer.

In a similar study, when participants were told only to check their steps if they wanted to, 71% later reported that they had checked regularly, even though they didn't have to. Humans are curious creatures, and if we know that number is there, most of us cannot resist the temptation to look at it, even if we couldn't care less when the tracker is off.

The same people who self-select to measure are those who are more likely to be hurt by it. People who wear pedometers walk further than those who don't wear them, but they also say walking feels more like work than pleasure, and report being less happy and satisfied at the end of the day. The potential harmful effects of tracking your activity go beyond just making the activity less enjoyable – excessively tracking can actually negatively affect your overall wellbeing.

So research shows that activity-tracking can decrease enjoyment of whatever form of movement someone is trying to measure and can even lead people to do less of it when they take the trackers off. One study, in 2017, found a link between the use of calorie-counting and/or fitness-tracking devices and eating disorder symptoms among college students. A survey of female Fitbit users undertaken in 2016 found that, although reaching the daily target led to feelings of self-satisfaction, almost 60% felt like their days were controlled by their devices, and 30% called the device an 'enemy' that made them feel guilty. I have heard people say that they feel their workout 'didn't count' because their tracker didn't register it properly. It definitely counts.

Food-diary apps like YouAte or YouFood are doing something new for dieting. These apps allow users to log meals and snacks, but where they differ from other measuring apps like MyFitnessPal is that they don't necessarily track calories. Instead, you're asked to categorise each meal as being 'on path' or 'off path'. YouFood in particular relies on images of food, so users don't have to weigh and count everything.

A food-diary app where you track using photos... doesn't that sound an awful lot like Instagram? Why, yes. Yes, it does. Instagram is a commonly used tool for people to track their food intake. Some people post food photos to Instagram to support their health goals, using it as an everyday tracking tool as they pursue healthy eating choices. Some do it to hold themselves accountable, whereas others see the tracking as a way to keep up their motivation.

Traditional methods for tracking food rely on pairing ingredients with calories or using a food scoring system such as the one employed by Slimming World. Apps like MyFitnessPal rely on food databases, which are often incredibly unreliable and inaccurate. They will contain standardised common food items like fruit and vegetables, but don't account for the variability in the food we eat. They often don't have nutritional information for meals eaten out (although most chain restaurants have this information online), and the time and effort it takes to weigh everything you're including in a recipe, means people can end up relying on prepared foods because the calories are right there on the packet. Recipes with fifteen ingredients made from scratch are such a hassle to track because, although you may know what's going in, the app doesn't account for nutrient availability changing during the cooking process. While you may be able to estimate you've eaten a quarter of whatever you've made, you don't know that each quarter has exactly the same ratio of ingredients – one portion may have more beans than another. This effort makes it harder for people to develop reliable, long-term tracking habits. It's tedious, and it's giving me a headache just thinking about it.

Often people choose Instagram because photo-based food tracking is seen as fun, easy and more social than traditional methods. It can also be used to motivate and encourage others to pursue health-orientated goals. Some want to build an audience and use their own health journey to inspire others, while also holding themselves accountable. We want to be able to do this on our own terms, though. In an online experiment, people were less willing to set themselves goals when they knew that announcements of their weekly physical activity goals would be posted automatically on Facebook. This was partly because of the public sense of accountability, and partly from a fear of cluttering friends' news feeds or appearing boring.

One of the big advantages of photo-based tracking is that images can help us access memories of that meal, where a list of ingredients and calories wouldn't have the same effect. Food photos feel closer to people's eating experiences. Plus, it's more socially acceptable to take a quick picture of your food for Instagram than it is to open up MyFitnessPal and start calculating everything before you start eating. A picture doesn't affect those around you anywhere near as much as tracking numbers, which can make others uncomfortable.

Another benefit of Instagram is that it helps people find community support. Many people find Instagram users more supportive than users of other social media platforms, which is understandable, as the idea of posting your daily food and workout to Facebook seems a bit strange. On Instagram people can choose to follow you, whereas on Facebook you're almost expected to befriend those you know in real life, regardless of whether or not you want to see what they have to say.

Instagram also provides a sense of motivation and accountability. Posting about accomplishments and goals reached means there's something to reflect and look back on when motivation is lacking, while also being used to motivate others. Some people find posting about bad days and difficult experiences helpful, as it leads others to reach out and offer emotional support. People are usually kind and will acknowledge you're trying. Some, however, find it uncomfortable to post about their failures or lapses because they don't want to disappoint others. They feel the need to justify their actions, for example explaining why they've gained weight or why they've had a 'bad' day of eating.

There is a desire to keep a public Instagram account interesting and engaging, which is a challenge when you're just posting the same thing every day - your food. This is why people often create two separate Instagram accounts: one for the food diary, and another for everyday life, to avoid oversharing and boring friends and family. The pressure to post something new and interesting each day can lead some people to take breaks from tracking, which then limits their ability to reflect back on past behaviour.

Tracking can also become obsessive and harmful. I went through a phase of tracking my food on MyFitnessPal once. It was miserable, and made me hate everything I was cooking and eating. I can honestly say my life was instantly better when I deleted that app forever.

Remember fitness blogger Tally Rye? She started getting into fitness at drama school, found the #fitspo* hashtags on social media, and joined Instagram to gain inspiration and motivation. She created an Instagram called @cleanfitlifestyle (which she cringes at now) and started posting fitness content. Tally would track her food intake, and post much of what she was eating on Instagram as a food diary. "I couldn't eat food without taking a picture of it, I had to post everything I made, and it all had to be Instagrammable – it had to be presentable and look a certain way."

While this started as a way to be healthier and hold herself accountable, Tally was feeling the pressure not just to look a certain way, but also to say "the right things". She says, "I'd say it was OK to go out and have fun and go out for dinner and eat whatever you want! But I knew that for me that happened so rarely and I would be thinking about that experience for a long time before and afterwards, and have to make up for it in other ways, like being super healthy with my food the next day or not skipping a workout."

Tracking her food and posting pictures of what she was eating became quite obsessive for Tally, and she remembers one clear example that illustrates how strict she was with herself: "There's a picture of me holding a single dark chocolate Lindt ball one Christmas, saying how I do allow myself to have treats at Christmas, which is actually really sad! Following other people who posted everything they ate in a day just validated my behaviours."

---

* #fitspo, also known as 'fitspiration' is a play on the word 'thinspiration' which is used on pro-anorexia sites. Fit + inspiration = fitspiration = fitspo for short.

Did Instagram enable and encourage this mindset? "100%. I had no exposure to nutrition information, my family never talked about diets at home, so all the information I initially got about nutrition was from social media – encouraging me to be gluten free and refined-sugar free and to eat clean." On top of that, Tally was surrounded by people online who were doing the same. "I used to follow all these people who were eating clean, tracking what they were eating, and posting the perfect breakfast every morning. I look back and I just think, wow, we were a bunch of very unwell people. Everyone stopped posting around 2016–17, and they must have stopped posting because it wasn't sustainable, or they had to seek treatment. Some of them, their last post was about how they're taking time away from Instagram for their mental health. Our disordered eating was really normalised and encouraged."

How does she feel now about the things she used to post? "I feel far removed from that person, but it also helps me understand and empathise with other people's approaches, views, and needs. I've never deleted anything I've posted. Someone recently commented on a post I wrote two years ago and asked me 'do you still believe this? You said something different the other day', and I said of course not, I'm an evolving human, and I have the right to evolve as much as anyone else."

Now, Tally rarely posts any food pictures on her social media accounts, which she says took time and wasn't an easy habit to get away from. "The main way I got past [having to take pictures of everything] was by deliberately making food that was really unattractive and messy so I couldn't justify photographing it."

Tally doesn't track her food anymore and doesn't recommend

it either. She says she's much happier now as a result, "because I'm not so preoccupied with food and my body."

Should you eat more mindfully?

Mindful eating is a non-judgemental awareness of physical and emotional sensations associated with eating. It involves:

- Slowing down the pace of eating, for example, by chewing more slowly, taking short breaks to assess how full you feel, or waiting until you've swallowed a mouthful before picking up the next item of food.
- Eating away from distractions such as driving or looking at screens.
- Using the body's hunger and fullness cues to inform the decision about when to start eating and when to stop.
- Acknowledging your own likes and dislikes from a place of curiosity, not judgement.
- Using all available senses when eating.
- Incorporating mindfulness practices as part of life.

Mindful eating is far more concerned with how we eat, rather than what we eat. Hopefully you can already see how social media can interfere with this process. We spend a considerable amount of time eating in front of screens – either our work computer, while watching TV, or while scrolling through social media. Mindful eating has risen in popularity in direct contrast to this increasing reliance on screens, our obsession with being busy, and our rising FOMO.

This isn't something we just do alone; more than a third of respondents to a UK survey said they sometimes or often use their phones when eating with family and friends.

When we eat and scroll/watch at the same time, we're distracted from our food, which makes it more difficult for us to determine how hungry we are, whether we enjoy the food, or when we're full. This means we're more likely to overeat, and research shows we often do. For example, in one study researchers investigated whether students would eat more while watching television: they ate 36% more pizza and 71% more mac and cheese while watching tv.

We know from research that screens tend to provide a stronger distraction than other activities like driving or eating with others, so people tend to eat more without even realising. I think many of us can relate to the idea of sitting in front of the TV with a bowl of popcorn, immersed in what we're watching, only to suddenly reach down and find the bowl empty. How did that happen? We're aware we've been eating, but not aware of the quantity. We're a little shocked, and might react by placing the bowl away and deliberately choosing not to make any more to eat, even if we don't feel full. Social media does, of course, require a little more interaction than watching TV, even if it's just scrolling with one thumb. Therefore, we may expect something as immersive as social media to have a stronger effect than television.

While distracted eating affects how much you eat in that moment, it also affects how much you eat later in the day too. In fact, distraction has an even greater effect on later eating than on immediate eating. This is likely because, when we are distracted, we don't lay down strong memories of the food, so that, hours later, our memories of how much we've eaten are hazy, and we eat more than we may need to. When we eat a meal mindfully and look back on it later in the day, we have a stronger concept of quantity, and therefore are able to make a more accurate judgement about how hungry we are and how much we need to eat.

Although in the moment we aren't aware of our less-than-mindful eating,* it's something we all recognise. We know that if we're scrolling on social media, watching one YouTube video after another, we don't pay as much attention to what we're eating. And, yet, we really struggle to stop doing this. One of the biggest barriers that prevents us from eating more mindfully is boredom. This can especially be the case if the food we're eating isn't particularly enjoyable – our phone becomes a welcome distraction from that disappointment. We can also easily become restless and get used to constantly multitasking, whether it's *needing* music while we're in the shower, listening to a podcast on the way to work, or using our phones while we eat. Finally, in a world where we prize efficiency and where being busy is seen as a sign of success, taking 20 minutes to simply eat and do nothing else feels either self-indulgent or a waste of time. I promise you it is neither of those things.

---

* Some researchers call this 'mindless eating' but I don't like this term, it's too absolute. It's not totally mindless, it's distracted eating. The term 'mindless eating' was coined by researcher Brian Wansink, whose research has since been discredited, which contributes to my preference here. The research cited in this section is, of course, not from his lab.

Photographed food is tasty food

Having said all this, there is a side of social media that can actually enhance mindful eating and help us develop healthier habits by being more conscious of what we're eating. Research suggests people eat less when they take photos of their meals, possibly because they're more mindful of what they're eating. That's right: taking pictures of your food might actually be a good thing. The very act of taking a picture before eating – searching for the right angle, the natural light, the slight tweaking of the positioning on a plate – can actually make food taste better.

The research looking into this included three linked studies. The first investigated the effects of photographing food before eating. Participants were assigned to one of four groups: take a picture of healthy food before eating it; just eat the healthy food; take a picture of indulgent food before eating it; or just eat the indulgent food. The indulgent food they were given was red velvet cake whereas the healthy one was a fruit salad. The results showed that those made to take a picture of red velvet cake perceived it to be tastier and more pleasurable than those who didn't take a picture of the exact same cake. There was no perceived difference in taste for those who photographed the healthy food compared to those who didn't.

For the second study, participants were given the same red velvet cake, but this time half were told it was indulgently made with all the traditional ingredients and cream-cheese frosting, whereas the other half were told it was healthy because it was made with applesauce, egg whites and low-fat frosting. Both groups were asked to photograph the cake before eating it.

Perhaps unsurprisingly, those who were told the cake was indulgent rated it higher than those who were told it was made with healthy ingredients. Having, in the past, made brownies with all manner of vegetable ingredients like sweet potato and beetroot, I can attest to the fact that if I'm now told the brownie I'm eating is a 'healthy' one, I don't like it. Screw vegetable cakes, give me butter and eggs all the way.

When we photograph our food, we end up delaying the part we're most excited about – the eating. We're anticipating the delicious flavours we're about to encounter, and as we saw in the introduction, the expectation of reward can be stronger than the reward itself. When you do eventually go to take that first bite, the food ends up tasting that much better.

This link between food photography and greater satisfaction explains why someone, once in the habit of taking food pictures, will automatically want to take their phone out at the dinner table. This habit can make an avid Instagrammer feel like something is missing if they don't perform this ritual.

This is consistent with a collection of studies published in 2013, which found that when people delayed eating by performing a short ritual of some sort, even if it was simple and mundane, it had a positive influence on how delicious they thought the food on their plate was. In one experiment, people were given a chocolate bar along with strict instructions on how to unwrap it before eating. Those people savoured the chocolate bar more and said they'd be willing to pay more than those who were just given a chocolate bar to enjoy with no ritual instructions. The short delay was key, but it only had a positive effect on the taste of the food if the behaviour was something repeated, fixed and relevant to the activity of eating. Simply waving the chocolate bar around for a minute wouldn't make any difference, but slowly unwrapping it would.

The idea of a repeated, fixed behavioural ritual describes the act of taking a food picture before eating perfectly: you take your phone out, open the camera app, position the plate and background, take a few pictures from different angles, take a quick look to make sure they're good, then put the phone away again. What enhances this further is the fact that there's often a sense of urgency – if the food is hot then taking too long will leave it cold and less enjoyable, if you're with others then you don't want to disturb them or piss them off with your photography. Most importantly, you actually want to eat and enjoy the wonderful food placed in front of you. In the end the ritual is still the same, and results in delayed gratification, and therefore more enjoyment of the food.

Of course, this can be taken too far, to the point where a dish that hasn't been photographed feels like a waste and doesn't produce the same level of satisfaction. The setting, the company, the venue... all these things matter as well as the food.

I want to add here that mindfulness can feel like just another thing you *have* to do and can add extra stress to your life. Mindfulness isn't something that requires spending money on silent yoga retreats or an expensive app – although if these are what are most helpful for you then by all means go for it – but is intended to be something that you spend a few minutes of time on, where you sit with your own thoughts and just exist.

If you're someone who has suffered trauma, mindfulness and meditation is not always something that's recommended, and can sometimes do more harm than good. In that case, I would recommend seeking help from a trauma-informed therapist who can guide you through a mindfulness practice and be there to support you if it brings up traumatic memories or a strong physiological response.

As with all things related to food, it's important to have a nuanced discussion around mindful eating.

How should you perform your eating?

I once went on a sort-of blogger trip to Bali.* One of the great advantages of going on group blogger trips is that everyone will want to take pictures of the food, which makes you feel more comfortable as you're not the only one doing it. After a couple of days, however, we noticed a trend. We'd go to a cafe, order a table full of delicious and beautiful food, and the servers would say to us: "Please, please eat the food!" The first few times we were a bit bemused, but reassured them we would, and then proceeded to eat everything in sight. Eventually we asked someone why they felt the need to tell us this, and the reply genuinely shocked me.

Apparently, it was very common for young, white bloggers to go to these restaurants, order a mountain of pretty food, take some pictures, pay, and just walk out. They'd order the food, and then not eat it. This was clearly common enough that it was causing concern at the amount of food waste being produced. I just couldn't understand why someone would not eat the food when it was so carefully prepared and arranged, and really did

---

* Don't worry, I hate myself more for that sentence than you ever could.

taste good (most of the time, at least). That has stayed with me ever since.

Now, with a far more cynical mind and the benefit of hindsight, I have a better understanding of why this happened, and still happens to this day. I'm still outraged, of course, but I can attempt to unpack it now.

Strangely enough, when researching this topic, I couldn't find anyone willing to admit to me that they had ordered food purely for photos and not for eating. The closest I found was what one blogger shared in an interview for *Food and Wine*: "When I first started my account, yes, I was eating everything. However, after a year or so, I gained probably 15 lbs so I decided I really had to cut back. I actually did [insert stupid fad diet] for a month to reset my system — for that month I didn't eat *any* of the food I posted."

There's something strange about seeing a bunch of thin and beautiful bloggers sharing pictures of large meals and yet their size or shape never changing. It's like a present-day version of socialite and heiress Paris Hilton from the early 2000s, who was famously photographed regularly with bags of fast food in her hand, all while remaining in an incredibly thin and toned body. It's a contradiction that's as compelling as the food itself: a beautiful woman constantly eating 'junk food', and yet never gaining weight. Paris Hilton was so good at exploiting the paradox of her body and her appetites that she booked an ad campaign where she holds a giant burger while wearing a very revealing swimsuit, sending a clear message that if you're cool enough the principles of thermodynamics don't apply to you.

Obviously, we all know that's not how bodies work, but it's still an irresistible fantasy. The idea of being able to eat everything you want without ever gaining weight is the ideal dream for so many people. Influencers and bloggers are often selling a fantasy, and admitting that they don't eat all the food they photograph would destroy that fantasy. This isn't so much the case for food bloggers, as their social media is more of a portfolio of their work, but lifestyle bloggers and fashion bloggers are, in essence, selling their life and lifestyle as their reality, as something aspirational. It can be hard to work out sometimes if their lifestyle really is 'real' or if it's something they aspire to as well.

This fantasy feels very different to me than knowing that food used in advertising is 'fake', for example that glue is used as a substitute for milk, or fake ice cream is made from vegetable shortening, powdered sugar and corn syrup. But these people posting images of food they haven't eaten are meant to be every-day people sharing their lives. It's supposed to be personal. Life-style, travel, food or fitness blogger... the food they're posting is part of the package that is them. The whole nature of it is supposed to be authentic.

(Not) Eating for the 'gram

Maxine Ali is a linguist and body-image researcher. When I asked her for her thoughts on performative eating she had a lot to say.

"Bloggers have made businesses out of sharing photogenic feasts, and restaurants have made it their niche to be crowned the most 'Instagrammable' foodie hotspot. Eating with our eyes is how the digital food-sphere thrives. So, it is perhaps telling that the one thing we never see in these images is the act of eating itself. The messy, carnal act of chewing, slurping and swallowing. Eating is only ever implied. A caption exclaiming

'OMG, best brunch ever', is enough to assure observing audiences that consumption has taken place, without being forced to confront the less aesthetically pleasing reality of actual, physical ingestion, the one aspect of food that is tinged with feelings of shame and indignation.

"Social media has a performative function. The images we choose to post are a process of self-creation, employed to construct meaning, share narratives, paint a desirable identity and participate in the practices of the communities we want to belong to. Food, as a symbol of morality, personality and affluence, becomes a tool through which we seek and attain social validation. In showcasing the kind of food cultures we dabble in online, by extension, we craft an idea of what kind of person we are, what kind of life we lead.

"Food porn doesn't always put on an authentic performance, however. It is often manipulated, manufactured to portray the most desirable version of oneself. For example, one might decide what to eat based on what kind of ingredients get the most engagement, or take photos of other people's meals to pass off as their own. Restaurant owners have even noticed a rising trend of diners ordering a feast's worth of dishes to get that perfect shot for Instagram, only [to] leave it all completely untouched. The ellipses of consumption has meant that eating is becoming further and further removed from the meaning and value we assign to food, to the point where it no longer even matters to the culinary experience.

"Under the new rules of identity according to social media, we are not what we eat, but rather what others believe we eat. It is society's impression of us that counts, not the pleasure and satisfaction we derive from eating what we like."

Challenge accepted

Ordering food and not eating it is one thing, but thanks to social media we've also seen a rise in performative eating, whereby people 'perform' eating challenges for the sole purpose of likes and shares.

YouTube inspires all sorts of ridiculous shenanigans and attention-seeking behaviour, and video challenges have been around for almost as long as the platform itself. Some of these, like the ALS Ice Bucket Challenge, are actually doing good. Others, however, are either totally ridiculous or downright dangerous, like the Cinnamon Challenge. One challenge in particular became famous in the wake of Olympic swimmer Michael Phelps revealing the huge quantities of food he eats while he's training: the 10,000 Calorie Challenge.* This is exactly what you'd expect: a YouTuber, usually young and thin, eats 10,000 calories worth of food in one day, and films the whole thing for entertainment value.

One of my main issues with this kind of challenge is that I don't think anyone would really do it if it was just for themselves, with no one watching it. It's done purely for validation from others.

This challenge is done predominantly by fitness bloggers who mainly post about their workouts and their #mealprep. This is unsurprising to me, because these people have made a name for themselves through messages of motivation, self-control and

* Others claim the trend started after Dwayne 'the Rock' Johnson started sharing 'epic cheat days' with his followers, including one on which he ate 12 pancakes, 21 brownies and 4 double dough pizzas. Impressive!

'staying on track'. By posting much of their everyday food and workouts, and by having a fit body, they are able to do this kind of challenge without any real criticism or health-shaming. Everyone watching knows that this is an exception to their disciplined life, and that they'll go straight back to that life once the challenge is over.

Many fitness bloggers, later in their online careers, will look back on their early days and admit their eating was disordered, that their body image was terrible, that their relationship with exercise was obsessive and unhealthy. For some, then, it seems this kind of extreme challenge is a controlled way of losing control, an excuse to carefully indulge all their food fantasies, to binge without being accused of having an eating disorder.

It's bizarre that we are happy to celebrate a fitspo eating 10,000 calories in one day for entertainment, when we'd express extreme concern if someone did this in private.

Fitness bloggers didn't invent this concept though. Eating a large number of calories in one sitting was first seen in South Korea, as part of the trend of mukbang videos. These videos involve a host surrounded by plates piled high with noodles or fried chicken or some other delicacy, who then eats this food while fans interact with them through a live chat and ask questions, which are answered live. Some viewers even offer payments in exchange for having some say in what the host eats next, or simply to say thank you.

The most popular videos are by young, thin women, again feeding into this fantasy of someone eating huge volumes of food and yet never gaining weight. Some people have actually generated a living from eating food online, and many YouTubers are picking up on this popular trend and creating their own eating videos. Millions of people watch these kinds of videos, but why? Why are we so fascinated with watching others eat?

Apparently, mukbangs originated in South Korea because of the growing number of single Koreans who feel alone and lonely, combined with the fact that eating is an inherently social aspect of Korean culture. While some fans of these videos simply crave the company of eating with someone else, even if it is through a screen, others use the videos to challenge and improve their own relationships with food. Some viewers feel they can satisfy their desire for food by watching others gorge on plates piled high. Others claim it helps them eat more as part of their eating disorder recovery process.

To be fair, there are arguably far worse challenges out there. The 10,000 Calorie Challenge, for example, isn't a significant health hazard. You're unlikely to suffer too much (other than feeling uncomfortable for a few hours). But there are other crazy challenges, like the Cinnamon Challenge, which can hurt the lungs if the cinnamon is inhaled, as easily happens. In 2015 a four-year-old boy died of asphyxiation after attempting this challenge. Then there's the Soy Sauce Challenge – which involves drinking scary amounts of soy sauce in one go – and that caused one 19-year-old to slip into a coma. He needed 6 litres of IV fluids to revive him.

Some people run marathons, some jump out of planes, others shovel a kilo of chicken wings into their faces just to have their photo displayed on the wall of their local diner, or to hit a million views. It seems we just really like watching people do extreme things that we either wish we could do or that we don't want to do but are intrigued by. I think it's the same reason why we enjoy watching the Olympic Games or have the Guinness

World Records. We're fascinated by the limits of what humans are capable of.

Please, sir, I want some more data

The idea that more data is always better doesn't stand up to scrutiny when it comes to health. Of course, it is very much down to individual preference, and if you're someone who finds benefit from trackers then please do continue. If, however, you're someone who finds it stressful and it makes you unhappy, then my recommendation would be to just stop. You do not have to track everything, or anything at all, in order to be healthy.

What the research into trackers shows is that we need to be mindful about *why* we are choosing to track aspects of our lives. It's not to suggest that no one should be tracking anything, but that we need to really assess whether we're doing this because we've been told it's a good idea, or whether we actually want/ need to know. If tracking your runs helps you stay motivated and keep progressing, then great! But maybe take the tracker off when you go out dancing, or when you're going for a walk while catching up with a friend.

Similarly, if you really enjoy watching people do crazy food challenges, don't let me stop you! I understand the fascination. But let's not encourage people to order mountains of food for the 'gram and then not eat it. We have enough of a problem with food waste around the world.

Finally, mindfulness and mindful eating is a great skill to learn, but it's not something you have to do at every meal to get the benefits. Sometimes you need to eat at your desk to get everything done, and sometimes you just want to eat a pizza on the sofa in front of the TV. That is totally OK. I would, however, recommend getting into the habit of leaving your phone in your bag or in another room while you're eating. You don't need to be scrolling – that can wait until after you're done.

3

HOW EXTREME
SHOULD I EAT?

Imagine you wanted to start a group, one that, let's say, revolved around a certain identity. Where would you do it? I bet you answered social media. Extreme groups take to social media because it's cheap, accessible and quickly reaches lots of people. The barriers are incredibly low, far lower than trying to share your ideology via a book, mainstream media, flyers, or finding a physical location in which to meet.

There are two forces that radicalise opinions in group discussions. One is informational: people learn new arguments to support the opinions they already hold. The other is social: people admire and want to emulate those expressing the most extreme opinions.

Discussions on social media carry both the informational and social forces of radicalisation. Tweets that offer new arguments supporting a particular attitude, whether it's useful, funny or just catchy, tend to get more likes and retweets because they capture our attention. This helps others to learn potential arguments or quips to reinforce their already-held beliefs. Individuals with more radical opinions also tend to get larger followings online, precisely because their tweets are polarising – those who agree will retweet, and those who disagree will quote tweet* explaining why, which links people back to the original tweeter. More radical individuals therefore end up with more social influence. Those in the middle tend to be perceived as boring in comparison.

Social media tends to be more radicalising than face-to-face groups because it produces larger collectives, which means more sources of information, and because the more people you have in a group the more likely you are to find extreme radicals. On top of that, radical extreme ideas can be more easily shut down in an in-person group, and you can kick people out for being too extreme. You can't do that online in the same way. Sure, you can hit the mute or block button, but that person can easily find a way round that.

Perhaps the most well-known example of social media-enabled extremism is the Red Pill men's rights activists.† Some young men find these far-right extreme videos by accident, others seek them out deliberately. Not everyone who views them ends up a neo-Nazi, but the risk is definitely there.

---

* While a retweet simply shares the original post as is, a quote tweet shares the post with your own additional comment alongside it.

† 'Red pill theory' is based on the movie *The Matrix* where the main character is offered a blue pill to stay plugged in where everything is nice and boring, or a red pill where he sees the world for how it really is. According to men's rights activists, the 'blue pill' is what women say they want from a man, whereas the 'red pill' is what, allegedly, women *really* want – which is to be dominated. Part of this thinking involves the idea that women owe men sex, and part of it is pure white supremacy.

Those who haven't deliberately sought out this kind of content will often share how they found them through YouTube and its recommendation algorithm. This is the software which determines what videos come up on your homepage as well as what is 'up next' when autoplay is on. According to YouTube, this algorithm is responsible for more than 70% of all time spent on the site – a stat they're proud of.

Of course, right-wing radicalisation of young men is driven by numerous complex factors, many of which have nothing to do with social media. But there's no denying that social media – and YouTube in particular – has created a dangerous slippery slope to extremism by combining two things: a business model that rewards provocative videos with exposure and advertising money, and an algorithm that guides users down paths designed to keep them glued to their screens for as long as possible.

The issue isn't just that videos claiming the moon landing was a hoax or that vaccines cause autism are found on YouTube. The massive library of videos is generated by users with little editorial oversight, as there are far too many videos for anyone to review before they appear online. This means misinformation is almost inevitable. The problem with YouTube is that it allows misinformation to flourish unchecked and, in some cases, through its powerful artificial intelligence system, it even provides the fuel that lets misinformation spread like wildfire.

Early in 2019, YouTube said it was working to change its recommendation algorithm to reduce the spread of misinformation and conspiracy theories. It's certainly capable of changing this – in its early days, YouTube noticed a sharp increase in pro-anorexia ('pro-ana') videos. It responded quickly, with moderators placing age restrictions on these videos, removing them from people's recommendations, or removing them from the platform entirely. It saw a trend in videos that threatened the health of its users and did something about it.

Since then, we have seen large numbers of anti-vaccine videos spread throughout the platform, which haven't been restricted or banned. With pro-ana content YouTube acted swiftly, so why isn't it doing the same for this public health crisis, which has now been named by the World Health Organisation as one of the ten threats to global health in 2019?

Somewhere between now and then, YouTube chose to prioritise chasing profits over the safety of its users. When you consider that every single day people watch more than one billion hours of YouTube content, that's a lot of videos.

As YouTube's system suggests more provocative videos to keep users watching, it can direct them towards extreme content they might otherwise never find or never would have considered searching for. The algorithm is designed to lead users to new topics to pique fresh interest. And it works.

YouTube is *the* platform for conspiracy theories. A search for 'Is the Earth flat or round?' yields an 80% support for the Earth being round on Google, but 90% support for flat-Earth theory on YouTube. Searching 'Is global warming real?' on YouTube provides recommendations that are 70% in favour of global warming being a 'hoax'. These conspiracies often use clever emotional tactics, which exist in stark contrast to the fact-based approach of science.

The algorithm is designed to promote maximum viewing time, and, let's face it, settled science often seems far more boring than wacky conspiracy theories. Consequently, the extreme pseudoscience gets more views, and is therefore promoted and recommended to other users so they too spend more time viewing. This way, pseudoscientific videos are pushed more by the algorithm than scientific ones, and it inadvertently encourages these ideas. YouTube benefits because the more videos we watch (and the more time we spend watching them), the more ads we see, and the more money YouTube can make.

Aside from the algorithms that hold incredible power of what we see, social media also amplifies ordinary social competition, which can drive people to extremes. You're no longer just competing with people around you, but with anyone, anywhere in the world. The way to make your videos go viral is to be the most extreme you can. This competition and risk-taking has led to a huge rise in what's known as 'death by selfie' – Wikipedia even has a list of people killed or nearly killed while trying to take selfies. Some are purely accidents, for example, one man tried to take a selfie with a bear and was sadly mauled to death, but others come from social media risk-takers, such as rooftoppers,* who fall from great heights to their deaths, with GoPro footage that never ends up making it onto the Internet.

Echo (echo, echo)

I've focused primarily on YouTube so far, because it differs from most other social media platforms in the way it recommends content to people, rather than recommending a person or an

---

* Rooftoppers climb as high as they can onto a building or tower and take pictures, often of their feet dangling over the edge.

account. But a phenomenon exists across social media that can also drive extremism: the echo chamber.

We know from systematic large-scale studies that holders of extreme views on social media don't tend to interact much with people outside their group and are more likely to engage with others who hold similarly extreme views. Those in the centre will engage more with a variety of views, even if these interactions aren't always positive. Echo chambers illustrate the idea that online conversations are typically divided into a variety of sub-groups, with people only talking to others with whom they are already in agreement. In these bubbles that people form online, extreme and outrageous views are not shut down but encouraged, without criticism. In echo chambers people end up only seeing their own views repeated back to them using slightly different words – it's a closed system, everyone singing from the same song sheet.

It may sound obvious that we prefer to engage with people we already agree with, because that's more comfortable, but there are some interesting theoretical explanations behind this. The most likely explanation is the human tendency towards 'homophily' – the tendency for people to seek out those who are similar to themselves. Because we tend to socialise with others who share similar characteristics, often termed social homophily, two people who are alike (or homophilous) are more likely to communicate well. As a result, exchange of information most frequently occurs between individuals who share some qualities. This tendency means that ideological fragmentation will naturally emerge, as a homophilous source is more likely to be perceived as credible, trustworthy and reliable.

Closely related to homophily is the idea of 'selective exposure', whereby people select information or sources they already agree with, while filtering out others. This is also known as confirmation bias. There is endless information on the Internet, but selective exposure means we will more readily enter into online discussions with people we already agree with, and ignore or unfollow those we disagree with. A small group of people may confront those with different views, but most of us are uncomfortable with that confrontation and prefer to remove it from our newsfeed.

In addition to this, people also have a tendency to modify their opinions to match what they perceive the group norm to be (see the discussion in chapter 1), or at least to keep quiet if they believe their views to be outside this norm. This mechanism means that existing groups tend to become more homogeneous over time, or, at the very least, give the illusion of being more similar. The potential anonymity offered by communicating online via social media may further enhance this process, as anonymity encourages a group mentality and 'de-individuation', which makes adopting group norms more likely.

We use social media to follow and engage with those we already agree with, to reinforce our views, rather than being exposed to those who would challenge them. This self-perpetuating cycle contributes to the onset and maintenance of ever-more extreme ideas.

Pushing towards the extreme

It's not just extreme politics and conspiracy theories that thrive online, it's health content as well. In an article for the *New York Times* in 2018, sociologist Zeynep Tufekci argues that YouTube is pushing more extreme content to generate clicks. Her examples included how videos about vegetarianism would lead to recommendations for videos on veganism, and ones about jogging would lead to recommendations about ultramarathons. She commented: "It seems as if you are never 'hardcore' enough for YouTube's recommendation algorithm." It promotes and recommends videos that constantly up the stakes to keep you engaged.

The quick, conversational nature of social media like Twitter and Instagram has made it incredibly easy to engage in real-time conversations with like-minded people, so it's not surprising that diet and fitness communities have sprung up around these platforms – you can post what you're eating and have ten people 'heart' the picture before you've even finished the last mouthful.

Social media is, in many ways, a pure democracy: anyone can upload pretty much anything they like and have their voice heard. No longer do we have to wait until the next diet book to find out what diet we should be following, we can just search online and find a young, slim, white, shiny human telling us all about what *they* eat, and therefore what they think you should eat too. In this way, social media has made everyone a potential expert.

Perhaps the key difference between dieting and food camps twenty years ago and now is the fact that we can have instant connection and gratification via social media. We are saturated with food images that have become more and more extreme. The most popular food-porn images and videos are of dishes that are almost impossible for a single person to eat. A burger isn't crazy enough, it has to be with several patties and mac and cheese, then deep-fried and served with a mountain of cheesy fries. Who cares for a picture of pizza when you can have a taco-stuffed crust pizza the size of your living room topped with fried chicken? You want your food to stand out? Make it as wild and extreme as you can. We are obsessed with the extreme, and that includes extreme diets. We love reading about Beyoncé's maple syrup cleanse – simply mix together maple syrup, water, lemon juice and cayenne pepper – or about people who claim to lose huge amounts of weight by only eating eggs. It fascinates us, especially when we can't imagine even giving it a try because it's that crazy. And yet over time we become so used to these crazy ideas that they begin to seem almost normal.*

There are around 100 million images uploaded to Instagram on a daily basis, and 720,000 hours of video on YouTube. That's more videos and images than anyone could possibly hope to view in several lifetimes. When we see hundreds or thousands of similar images/videos, inevitably the ones that will grab our attention will be the weird and wonderful and extreme. These will stand out. The algorithms in place only enable a behaviour that's already built into our brains: the seeking out of the novel and exciting. If we scroll past hundreds of images of bowls of pasta, the one that's bright green is going to jump out, or the one that's piled so high we can't possibly imagine finishing it. In this way, both our brains and the algorithms on social media nudge us in the direction of more extreme content online.

On top of this, people love having their ego stroked, and the idea that their crazy way of eating is something only done by the select few 'enlightened' makes them feel special. Sprinkle with a little conspiracy theory (if you're low-carb, it's that fibre

---

* Obviously, please don't try any of these things at home. As a health-care professional I would never dream of recommending something so extreme to anyone.

isn't important; if you're vegan, it's that the meat lobby is all-powerful), place in an echo chamber, and you have an instant recipe for feeling superior. Open your eyes, sheeple!

Combine the egotistical aspect of human nature with the amount of time we spend online, and the low barrier for entry social media has (throw in a nice absence of fact-checking for good measure), and you create a perfect environment for conspiracy theories to thrive in, and the most restrictive eating patterns to build large communities.

I've seen this on my own Instagram too. Back in the day when my account was solely about sharing food, anything that was tagged #vegan was far more popular than #vegetarian, and #rawvegan usually received even more likes. The more extreme the food in the image, the more people engaged with that photo. My most popular food photos were never the most delicious, they were the giant fruit platters or huge bowls of raw salad vegetables. Extreme in quantity and extreme in ideology.

Kimberley Wilson is a chartered psychologist and offers up some really insightful explanations as to why extremism thrives on social media. "I think it's a combination of factors. First of which is the algorithm, the way that platforms are set up to bring you more of the things you 'like' or have already interacted with. 'Because you follow'. 'You liked a post tagged...'. A few clicks and you've gone from reading one meat-free recipe to misinformation about what causes cancer and conspiracy theories about how researchers are colluding to keep people sick and suppress 'natural knowledge'. It takes very little effort on the user's part to end up in very extreme corners of social media.

"This combines with our innate psychology – our tendency to view information that corresponds to our extant beliefs as 'facts' and conflicting information as false. So not only are we more likely to *look for* information that confirms our beliefs, but we also *interpret* new information to fit our pre-existing worldview."

This phenomenon is also known as confirmation bias – if you ask Google a question then the first link you select is far more likely to be one that sounds like what you want the answer to be, or what you already believe. For example, you could search 'does dairy cause cancer?' and find two links, one directly above the other, which say, 'Dairy Causes Cancer' and 'Dairy Doesn't Cause Cancer'. People will choose the one that confirms what they want to believe. This is a logical fallacy that we all commit sometimes, simply because we're human.

"Finally, the consistency principle means that we don't like to appear inconsistent in our ideas or behaviours." Kimberley observes, "This can be useful if you are trying to build a healthy habit (like committing to flossing everyday) as it can help improve adherence. The problem is that social media creates a *permanent record* of previous activities. This makes it very difficult to appear to change your mind (even if you do so in the light of new/better evidence). So, people end up feeling compelled to remain on the same track, even if that track starts to feel extreme or no longer right for them, in order to appear consistent to their prior position and avoid criticism from others of 'selling out' or being 'fake'. You see the same in politics. Whereas we should be commending people for updating their ideas once in possession of better evidence, they instead are criticised for making a 'U-turn'. This kind of condemnation of thoughtful re-evaluation of one's position is actually the opposite of what we encourage for good mental health."

Particularly if you're part of an online food and health community, rejecting that extreme food ideology also means rejecting those people you connected with, which makes it all the more difficult to change your mind, even if you recognise this way of eating isn't the right way for you, or is too extreme for you.

Extremes at both ends: From fruitarian to carnivore

Not that long ago, veganism was considered an extreme way of eating. Only a few years back, vegans were thought to be malnourished, self-righteous, sandal-wearing, bearded, tree-hugging, animal-cuddling, rabbit-food-eating hippies. Now veganism has gone mainstream, and isn't considered extreme at all, but borderline necessary by many. It's led to the rise in flexitarians and plant-based eaters, both of whom adopt a 'part-time vegan' approach that's designed to be more approachable.

Since veganism is no longer considered extreme, more restricted forms of eating have emerged to take its place. In recent years we have seen a rise in popularity in uber-extreme diets: from raw veganism to fruitarians, ketogenic to carnivores. It's impossible to ignore the role that social media has played in making these diets more accessible.

Self-styled health and wellness gurus have taken social media as their platform of choice for spreading the gospel about their eating habits. Slimming World and Atkins are so 'been there done that' – the new place to find what diet you should try next is YouTube, sometimes Instagram, or even Twitter. There are a number of more extreme and unusual ways of eating that have social media to thank for a considerable proportion of their popularity, so let's examine a few of these. I've placed these in a very particular order, adopting a fairly chronological timeline.

Paleo

This is an attempt at recreating the diet of humans living in the Paleolithic era, which is why it's also known as the caveman diet. The idea behind it is that our health has been declining since we started farming (it hasn't), that modern technology is making us all sick (the opposite, actually), and that our genes haven't changed since we were cavemen (they have), therefore, for optimum health, we should return to eating how we did back in the Old Stone Age. Slight problem though: there is no one accurate paleo diet. What Paleolithic-era humans ate depends on exactly which dates of the Stone Age you're looking at (it spans over 2 million years) and which part of the globe (different land masses yielded very different kinds of foods). In reality, these inconveniences are ignored, and a blanket guideline of anything pre-agricultural goes. Which means no grains, beans, potatoes, dairy, sugar, or anything that's considered 'processed'. This leaves you with meat, fish, eggs, nuts, seeds, vegetables and some fruit. Ironically, it also rewards you with paleo fruit and nut bars, which are most definitely processed. Paleo's popularity really kicked off in 2000, but saw a big spike from 2010 onwards, in particular on Instagram, directly parallel to the rise in veganism. #paleo has been used on Instagram over 14 million times.

Paleo was the hardest of these different diets to allocate to a particular social media channel. Low-carb diets tend to do well on Twitter, and variations of veganism on Instagram, but paleo seems to defy that trend. Thankfully, the writer and linguist Maxine Ali has a beautiful explanation: "From an ideological standpoint, [paleo] is very primal, almost anti-intellectualism because it's like going back to our instinct before science and technology started corrupting nature. So perhaps an image-based platform [like Instagram] fits perfectly, because it's more symbols and signs – rudimentary communication." Instagram as a modern form of cave painting. Now that makes sense to me.

Raw veganism

Raw vegans only eat plant foods, and nothing heated above 40°C (roughly 104°F). This naturally makes it much stricter than veganism, and also excludes potatoes, beans and lentils, which are either inedible or harmful when eaten raw. The most famous examples on YouTube would be Fully Raw Kristina (real name Kristina Carrillo Bucaram, who I used to follow... wow), and Freelee the Banana Girl (real name Leanne Ratcliffe). Freelee quickly rose to online fame when she made videos of herself eating 30 bananas in one day. The raw vegan community is full of misinformation, and there are some crazy claims made by the likes of Kristina about how eating raw vegan changes your eye colour to blue, which has some freaky elements of eugenics about it. For some reason that weirds me out more than the claims of curing cancer (it doesn't). Freelee also made a video saying, "I still believe that, largely, menstruation is toxicity leaving the body... So a lot of people are having these heavy, heavy periods and painful periods because they have a toxic body or have a toxic diet." Crazy, but she's not the only one. Miliany Bonet, on her blog RawVeganLiving, wrote a post stating that menstruation is a sign of a 'highly toxic' diet and lifestyle. She wrote: "If there is nothing to clean, there's no reason to menstruate," insinuating that by eating a 'clean' raw vegan diet your body is so clean you no longer need periods. Obviously, this is totally batshit crazy and wrong on so many levels. Periods are not 'toxic', they are a part of normal human functioning, and losing your periods is often a sign that something is wrong, not that you're doing something right.

What I find particularly interesting about this is how much it highlights the female domination in vegan and raw vegan spaces. More on that later. Raw veganism owes its popularity largely to YouTube, and partly to Instagram, as this diet is very heavy on fruit with some vegetables, and as such tends to be very colourful – making it ideal for a visual medium.

Keto

The ketogenic diet first appeared as a medical intervention for treatment-resistant forms of epilepsy. Now it's used mainly as a weight-loss diet. The idea behind keto is this: your body's preferred energy source is carbohydrates, as pretty much every single cell in your body can use glucose for energy. If you don't consume enough carbohydrates, and you use up your body's glycogen (carbohydrate chains) stores, your body flips a switch and enters a state known as ketosis. In this state, your body uses alternative energy sources such as dietary fat and converts them to carbohydrate-like substances called ketones. This is necessary for survival as your brain can't directly use fat or protein for energy. So, to ensure you don't starve your brain of fuel, your body undergoes this change, which it immediately flips out of if you eat the equivalent amount of carbohydrates found in a slice or two of bread. In order to stay in ketosis you have to consume a very high-fat, reasonably high-protein, ultra low-carb diet. All grains, starchy vegetables, sugar, beans and lentils are off the table, as is most fruit.

Like most diets on the low-carb side, keto has drawn a large crowd on Twitter, perhaps because it is less visually appealing and more male-dominated. Twitter is awash with anecdotes from men who are so secure in themselves they will make fun of your name and ask 'do you even lift?' rather than debate the science with you (true story). Whereas raw vegans on Instagram rely more on 'look how pretty this food looks, I'm eating so much, it's not restrictive at all!', keto advocates favour the written word. Instead of pictures of food, there is a huge reliance on before-and-after photos, and (more commonly) unsolicited written testimonials. Keto, unlike raw veganism, acknowledges that it's restrictive and has more of a 'no pain no gain' vibe, which is far more suited to Twitter than Instagram.

Fruitarian

Being a fruitarian means eating nothing but fruit, with perhaps a sprinkling of nuts and seeds if you feel like it. Most famously, the late Steve Jobs, CEO of Apple, spent some time as a fruitarian, which he claimed fuelled his creativity. But when actor Ashton Kutcher tried to follow a fruitarian diet for a month while preparing to play Steve Jobs in a film, he ended up in hospital. Some people in the community even go so far as to recommend 'mono meals', where you eat nothing but one single food (often bananas or watermelon) for a day or several days on end, which is supposed to 'cleanse' the system.

As part of my research for this chapter, I watched some videos on the Woodstock Fruit Festival on YouTube, and even I, as someone who dabbled in raw veganism and *suffered*, was slightly tempted by how happy, beautiful and free all the people looked, and how delicious the food seemed. It's brilliantly promoted as being so aspirational that you can't help but think 'maybe I could/should do that?' Don't panic, dear reader, I snapped out of it pretty quickly.

Carnivore

Or as I prefer to call it, the Jordan Peterson Meat and Misogyny Diet. This is the diet employed by incels* who find feminism and equality so frightening they have to make themselves feel more manly by eating meat. All the meat. All day, every day. The two major players in this field are Shawn Baker, a former orthopaedic surgeon from California who had his licence revoked and is known online as the 'carnivore king', and Jordan Peterson, Canadian professor of psychology who apparently can't tell the difference between a human and a lobster. Peterson got the idea from his daughter Mikhaila, who talks about how wonderful this diet has been for healing her chronic autoimmune

---

* Incels are 'involuntary celibates' – a group of men who are unable to find a partner despite wanting to, and who blame women for their lack of sexual intimacy. In extreme cases, they want to shame and physically harm women for not sleeping with them. There have been several documented cases where incels have become mass shooters or have driven their car into pedestrians, killing several people.

problems (for now) and sells individual consultations despite a complete lack of qualifications. I'm slightly confused as to why consultations would be needed. 'Hey, I'm looking to follow a carnivore diet, please help,' 'Just eat meat. That'll be $120 please.' Mikhaila now calls her eating pattern The Lion Diet and for $599 per year you can sign up for live videos and receive invites to meet-ups to discuss just how much meat you're eating. In defence of carnivores, apparently some of them also eat eggs and salmon, which somehow makes it... OK?

It goes without saying that this is probably the worst diet in existence, as we humans are omnivores and cannot produce certain nutrients, such as vitamins, which instead we have to obtain from food, often from plants. Vitamin C, for example, is an essential nutrient that is found in many fruits and vegetables. Sailors used to develop scurvy – a disease resulting from vitamin C deficiency – after long journeys at sea. The only reason I can think of why the Petersons don't have scurvy yet is because humans can obtain some vitamin C from raw organ meat, which doesn't sound particularly pleasant. A Scottish surgeon in the Royal Navy, James Lind, is generally credited with proving that scurvy can be successfully treated by eating citrus fruit in the 1700s. So we've known since the mid-eighteenth century that humans suffer without fruits and vegetables in their diet, but apparently feminism is just that frightening.

You think I'm joking, but not only do we have clear examples of the language used in the carnivore community ('soy boy' to describe men who don't eat meat and therefore must be more feminine), we also have the general misogynistic and right-wing views espoused by one of its leaders, Jordan Peterson, firm favourite among neo-Nazis and incels, as well as research showing that people who have very strong positive views about eating meat are more likely to hold sexist views. This is all without even delving into the fact that the carnivore community thrives on Reddit, the same platform that remains popular among said incels. If you think Mikhaila Peterson being female doesn't fit in this argument, I invite you to check out her Instagram, which is essentially a place for her to post thirst traps for all the old men who tell her she's beautiful. Did someone say internalised misogyny?

The pendulum swing

With these last two dietary patterns in particular, the most extreme versions of high- and low-carb eating, I can imagine it would be almost impossible to find someone within your friendship group who eats the same way. Social media is one of the few places where you're likely to easily find someone who eats the same way as you, even if that way of eating is batshit crazy. Extreme forms of eating have existed for a long time, but before social media people weren't able to share this aspect of their lives with so many people so easily, which is why such diets never spread in the same way they do today. Now, it doesn't matter if none of your friends eat the same way as you, because you can find online friends who do.

The overall pattern seems to be this: imagine a pendulum swinging from one side to another. On the one side we have higher-carb, plant-focused ways of eating, and on the other we have lower-carb, animal-heavy diets. We don't have to start with paleo, we can go as far back as vegetarianism, swinging over to

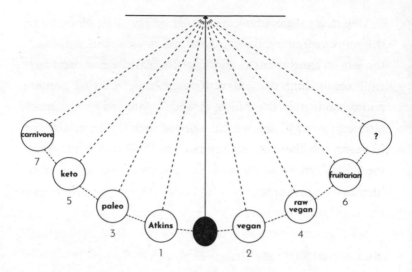

The chronological pendulum swing of extreme eating.

Atkins, then back, and higher, to veganism, across higher still to paleo, then raw veganism, keto, fruitarianism, and the carnivore diet. Each pendulum swing takes momentum from the previous, and takes it higher, to further extremes. The stronger the swing on one side, the stronger the response on the other.

Based on this pattern, if I had to predict what will come next, I reckon it would be something like the Rice Diet. Either eating nothing but rice, or something similar, that will be very high-carb and focuses around one particular food, similar to the carnivore diet. Either that, or perhaps the carnivore diet is the pinnacle of bullshit food extremism that privileged humans can reach and the pendulum will drop down and start over. I kind of hope that it's the second scenario.

What's also interesting about this is that you'll generally find the more extreme the diet, the stronger the gender divide. To the left on the low-carb end its predominantly men, and to the right on the high-carb, plant-focused end you'll find predominantly women. In the middle it tends to be a little more mixed, although you will still see far more women than men dabbling in veganism. There are several reasons for this, but a lot of it is rooted in how we use food to perform gender (meat = masculine, salad = feminine), and also that Instagram is more popular among women than men.

It's also important to acknowledge that these extreme diets can be incredibly expensive. Eating nothing but rib-eye steak is not cheap, and ensuring your fruitarian diet isn't boring by eating a variety of exotic fruit can get costly quickly. Add onto that the supplements you may need to take to get everything you're missing out on and you have a very expensive way of eating that few can afford. Those in the US may claim it's cheaper than healthcare, and they could be right. In the UK where healthcare is free... not so much.

'This food will cure every problem under the sun'

Of course, it's not just whole dietary patterns that can be extreme; food extremism has risen on social media in the form of 'miracle foods' such as celery juice. I write about many topics on Instagram that could be seen by some as 'controversial'. Personally, I don't see correcting misinformation as controversial, but when it's a divisive subject like food, people can become defensive very quickly, and take it as a personal attack.* I receive abuse and nasty messages on social media on a weekly basis, but never have I had so much hate directed at me as the time I wrote about celery juice.

The reason half of Hollywood and two-thirds of Instagram was drinking celery juice every morning in 2019 was because of one man: the Medical Medium. Anthony William is a man who has precisely zero qualifications in anything to do with food and health, instead he gets his wisdom from a spirit from the future who tells him, 'the secret to life, the universe and everything is celery juice!' (I'm paraphrasing, but you get the idea). He claims that celery juice can cure pretty much everything under the sun. Acne? Celery juice! Diabetes? Celery juice! Cancer? Celery juice! There's a hilarious yet disturbing video online where he meets one of the Kardashians (honestly I can't tell them apart anymore), and waves his hands all over her in a really awkward way, then proclaims her problems lie in her liver (it's always the fucking liver with him) and recommends... you guessed it: celery juice! He's an absolutely massive quack, truly one of the kings of quackery. When I wrote about celery juice on Instagram, I knew it would potentially cause some strong emotions to come forward, so I didn't even bother writing about how celery juice doesn't do anything, how any benefits people feel are likely due to the placebo effect, changing other parts of their diet, or the fact that they're more hydrated. I simply said: "Are we sure we want to take health advice from someone with no qualifications who talks to spirits? Isn't that a bit concerning? Oh, and anecdotes

---

*   If you're interested in this topic, I spend most of *The No Need to Diet Book* examining why humans have such a weird relationship with food.

aren't good enough science, otherwise we'd have to bring back exorcism and drinking your own urine on the National Health Service (which would obviously be a terrible idea)." I thought this was reasonable. But whenever my faith in humanity reaches a certain height, Instagram knows just how to shit all over it, and boy did it. I lost over 1,000 followers overnight and received so much abuse I had to switch off comments and DMs for more than 24 hours. At the time it was quite disheartening, but now, with hindsight, I find it fascinating just how angry people were about it. Up until that point these people had been very happy for me to tell them how 'detoxes' were a load of rubbish, how 'superfood' isn't a scientific term, and dairy doesn't cause cancer, but this was too far.

Miracle foods in some shape or form are incredibly popular on social media, as the succinct nature of 'cures all' fits very well into a 280 character limit, or as a soundbite to grab someone's attention. I know how hard it is to create a snappy infographic for Instagram that accurately portrays a nuanced topic and invites people to read more. With miracle foods, that job is so easy.

A 'miracle' is defined as 'an extraordinary and welcome event that is not explicable by natural or scientific laws', so let me start by saying food absolutely obeys natural and scientific laws. Vague sciency-sounding claims such as 'boosts cognitive function', 'balances your hormones', 'cleanses the liver', are effective marketing terms that often simply mean 'take this and your body will keep doing what it's doing anyway' – which sounds far less exciting.

Whether it's chia seeds, coconut oil, goji berries, apple cider vinegar, spirulina or celery juice, we love the idea of a simple 'miracle' cure or ingredient that we can eat to achieve perfect health, and social media is an incredible enabler of these kinds of claims.

The idea of specific foods curing specific conditions doesn't stand up to scrutiny. It would be wonderful if it were true, of course, but food isn't medicine. Unless you have an allergy, one food simply doesn't have that much power over you, although Instagram would say otherwise.

The prevailing power of anecdotes

On social media anecdote is king, and sharing your personal story is seen as empowering even if it's full of dangerous mis-information that can harm others. Saying 'this food cures cancer' is illegal under the Cancer Act of 1939, but saying 'eating this cured my cancer' is a lot more dubious.

Justin Stebbing, a consultant oncologist and professor of cancer medicine and oncology at Imperial College London, said in a 2015 interview for the *Guardian*: "As a patient, disease makes you lose control. People immediately want to regain that control and a very easy way for them to do that is by diet, and they can get all sorts of things off the Internet. We should understand that the Internet is a double-edged sword and if we're looking for information we should go to reputable sites."

Sasha* was diagnosed with Crohn's disease when she was 21. She recalls: "I had been unwell for some time before this but like a lot of people the condition went undiagnosed and it wasn't until I was admitted to A&E as an emergency that the diagnosis

* Name changed.

was made. It's an autoimmune condition that affects primarily the digestive tract but can manifest itself in other parts of the body (e.g. joints, eyes, skin) and also more generally as fatigue. I've spent two periods of time in hospital as a result of quite severe flare-ups of the condition that have required blood transfusions and IV steroids but now have the condition quite well controlled thanks to being on some of the newer biologic drugs in addition to the more standard immunosuppressants. I undergo regular blood tests and hospital visits to monitor the condition. I have to be careful what I eat as high fat or very fibrous foods can be very difficult to digest."

As a result of her diagnosis, Sasha found food both incredibly stressful and something she desperately wanted to have control over. She explained: "In between invasive medical procedures, medication and having to take me away from university, it was the only thing I could control in my life and about my body. I think the clean-eating craze tapped into my need to control my body again and gave me an excuse to justify this control because I was being 'healthy'. It allowed me to justify behaviours that had previously been identified as damaging (restrictive calorie control, selective eating and exclusion of food groups) under the banner of 'clean eating'. Around this time, there was also a number of individuals appearing on social media who were claiming miraculous recoveries from autoimmune conditions."

Sasha gives Instagram a lot of credit for her food obsession: "Looking back on this time I realise that Instagram is an easy place for people with any form of disordered eating to find validation in their behaviours – there are endless posts, endless photographs and endless 'miracle cure' stories that I think I would have struggled to find in mainstream media. There is another layer of validation provided within the Instagram community through likes and comments on posts that made the posts seem more important perhaps than an article that appeared in a magazine. The accessibility of the information and the highly visual nature of the information, I think, was also a critical part of the appeal of Instagram and how it reinforced my feelings. I don't think print media would have had the same effect as it is less immersive."

When I asked her what she would say to the people who influenced her diet, her answer both saddened and angered me. "It's hard to put into words – I'd really like to convey all of the rage and hurt that I still feel about having been so miserable and what could arguably be considered as being made so mentally unwell through disordered and dangerous eating practices that I only developed through exposure to Instagram! The effect will never go away, it can only be managed."

Sasha isn't alone with her story. I have heard hundreds like hers over the years via social media. These extreme ways of eating can drive us to judge and shame each other's food choices, as we'll see in the next chapter.

4

WHY ARE WE FOOD SHAMING EACH OTHER?

In early 2019, famous YouTuber Rawvana was caught eating fish in a video, which ignited a huge scandal in the vegan community. Rawvana (real name Yovana Mendoza) had made her name as a vegan influencer, posting videos about the vegan food she ate and selling plans to help others go on raw food 'cleanses'. The backlash was swift and severe. Followers flooded the comments section of her Instagram posts with the fish emoji, and the vegan YouTube community created video after video, discussing the drama and feeding the frenzy. A quick trip down the vegan rabbit hole on YouTube reveals a community that is rife with gossip and 'diss' videos that criticise and judge other creators' personalities, diets, exercise habits and, of course, appearance. They were having a field day.

Yovana made a video to explain her side of the story, claiming that she had dealt with a number of health-related issues, and was recommended by doctors to reintroduce animal products into her diet. Although she struggled to accept this, she did, and quickly her health started to improve. Despite this explanation, she was accused of lying to her fans, as she was apparently promoting her vegan e-Books while secretly struggling, and still posted vegan videos even after she had seemingly stopped being vegan. She had close to half a million subscribers, and many of them felt deceived and outraged, accusing her of animal cruelty, of being a fraud, selfish, of profiting from the vegan movement. Over 30,000 people unsubscribed from her channel in the first 48 hours. In response to this, she took a 4-month break from posting on YouTube, then returned with a number of videos explaining the process of breaking away from veganism, as well as how she doesn't label her diet anymore. Her Instagram is going strong with over a million followers, some of whom are still asking "I thought you were vegan?" over a year later. The YouTube outrage continues, with many still calling her a fraud.

Yovana is not a one-off. Other vegan YouTubers have come out and declared they are no longer vegan, including Bonny Rebecca and Tim Shieff. Tim decided to leave the platform after admitting he ate eggs and salmon after a 35-day water fast (water fasts are a terrible idea, please don't do them). He claimed he had experienced a number of health problems on a vegan diet, including "digestive issues, depression, fatigue, brain fog, lack of energy", and that it caused him "a huge identity crisis" to eat animal products again.

As a result of all this, articles have been written and videos have been made about how vegan YouTube is 'imploding'. These people are not vegan celebrities, they are celebrity vegans, people who have become famous online simply for being vegan, and as such their entire online persona is based around veganism. What does a celebrity vegan do when they're no longer vegan?

The criticism and food shaming that has been thrown at these individuals has come almost entirely from other vegans. People are incredibly angry and feel betrayed. But why does this elicit such a strong and hateful response from a community that prides itself on compassion? The people who seem the most upset are the ones who have been subscribers the longest, and those who have handed over money in exchange for the plans and eBooks that promise to help you achieve your vegan dreams, whether it's weight loss, clearer skin, a flatter stomach, detoxing or better energy. People feel they have invested considerable time and energy in supporting these individuals, and when they turn around and say 'I've changed', it feels like a slap in the face, because they *owe* them better. They feel their investment hasn't paid off, that they've been lied to, and so they lash out. There is a misconception that vegans who become unwell simply didn't 'do veganism' correctly, which is incredibly harmful. But people would rather believe that they had just done it wrong, rather than it *being* wrong. On some level I find this very understandable, although absolutely not to the point where it results in sending abusive messages. I can understand the disappointment, as I'm sure many of us have felt it at some point or another, when we heard the allegations against Kevin Spacey, or saw Beyoncé's incredibly restrictive post-baby diet that she shared in her Coachella documentary while simultaneously preaching self-love and self-acceptance. We invest our time and money in these celebrities, and in return we expect perfection, consistently. But, of course, this is unrealistic.

Social media allows us to share curated snapshots of our lives. Everybody filters their life online to a certain degree, and everyone shows a more idealistic version of themselves, because social media allows you to place an aspirational filter over your life. Followers and subscribers take this at face value, and fill in any gaps with more of the same.

One of the more harmful outcomes of the increasingly tribal nature of food online is an increase in food shaming. Food shaming is the unhealthy practice of criticising others' food choices based on self-prescribed parameters of what is a 'good' or 'right' choice. In this way, food shaming is intrinsically linked to the idea that your food choice is a proxy for your worth as a human being.

The pressure to make certain food decisions to prove yourself or to showcase yourself in a certain light is very real. There is a pressure to eat 'healthy' foods and make sure people see you're looking after your health, and equally there's a pressure to eat 'fun' foods – otherwise you're boring. Enjoying these 'fun' foods is part of being an ultra-desirable 'cool girl', an archetype that author Gillian Flynn describes in her bestseller *Gone Girl* as someone who "jams hot dogs and hamburgers into her mouth like she's hosting the world's biggest culinary gang bang while somehow maintaining a size 2."

But social media plays by different rules. When people do eat these 'fun' foods online, they are still shamed. In 2014, a commuter noticed that it was far more common for women to eat on the London Underground than men. For some reason, in response to this observation, he decided to form a Facebook group called Women Who Eat on Tubes. He invited people to take photos of these women, without them noticing, and post them in his group. The group grew quickly – at one point it had over 24,000 members – and people started mocking and shaming the women in the photos. The women were different shapes and sizes, and eating a variety of foods, but all were shamed. The issue wasn't so much what they were eating, but that they were eating in public in the first place. In response, women across London staged an 'eat-in' called Women Who Eat Wherever the Fuck They Want.

A few years back, someone created an Instagram account called 'You Did Not Eat That' (YDNET), which was dedicated to calling out women who post pictures of themselves looking like thin, toned models (which they often are), holding food that they apparently can't possibly have eaten because they're thin. Some of the photos that have been shared on this account are of models on photoshoots who are clearly just doing what they've been paid to do: posing for a photographer.

It's really yet another attempt to police women's behaviour, and make assumptions about people simply based on the way they look. Rather than speaking some kind of truth about women and food, it sends a clear message: as a woman, your body and your appetite are public property and fair game for comment, instruction and policing.

To caption a photograph of someone eating crisps with 'On Tuesdays we pretend to eat Cheetos' is mean and unnecessary. It implies two things: first, that these women are lying about what they eat, and second, that only fat people eat crisps, which is completely untrue.

I can understand the frustration behind an account like YDNET, as social media feels so curated, and people exaggerate, lie or omit things all the time. That's part of the appeal in the first place. So of course people lie online about what they eat. There's also a huge double-standard where thin women are often allowed to show themselves eating whatever they want like it's a personality trait, whereas fat women would be vilified for eating almost anything. But this frustration and these attacks are heavily skewed towards attacking women.

Why?

The better question is this: why do these women (not the models, of course) feel the need to post alongside these foods in the first place? Maybe they are eating the foods, that's a very real possibility, but regardless, it seems like they're normalising themselves. "Hey, I eat doughnuts too!" or possibly, "I can eat doughnuts and still look like this, sucks to be you!"

Top Chef host Padma Lakshmi bluntly calls the obsession with women's liberated eating habits "a male fantasy", telling the *New York Times*, "Look, the two things we need to survive in life are food and sex or love. Food for our bodies, and love for our hearts. So what is better than the archetypical image of a woman eating succulent, dripping, greasy, comforting food?"

These ideas have seeped so far into our consciousness, I can't count how many times I have heard smart, successful, kind, incredible women feel they have to justify eating something that could be seen as indulgent. "Oh, I'm only getting a second slice of cake because I went to the gym earlier", or "I'm allowing myself this treat today, I've been so good all week", or "I don't normally eat like this, I'll work it off tomorrow." Entirely unsolicited, and in a self-deprecating tone that aims to ward off any criticism. After all, by shaming ourselves first we are attempting to take that power away from others.

Indulgent foods like cake are damn delicious. The size of the slice on your plate, the number of slices of cake, how much exercise you've done, what else you've eaten... all these things should be completely irrelevant. And yet, so many intelligent and otherwise confident people feel the need to pre-empt judgement about their eating.

So why do we indulge in food shaming? Why are we so quick to judge others by their food choices, both on and offline? There are a number of potential reasons:

1. You are what you eat

Just think about how many online quizzes you've done that will tell you what your next partner will be like, or where you should live, depending on what your favourite cheese or ice cream flavour is. We so firmly believe that everyone's food choices say something about them. One study found that almost three-quarters of people believe that the contents of someone's shopping trolley sends a powerful message about that person. Interestingly, algorithms are doing exactly this with the data from our supermarket shops. Apparently, the most significant item that gives you away as a responsible, house-proud individual more than any other purchase is fresh fennel.

We will also make decisions about what to eat based on the impression and identity we want to portray to others, and we expect others are doing the same, as discussed in chapter 1. When food and eating is a form of identity, any kind of perceived attack on the food we eat becomes an attack on ourselves, and we retaliate with anger, choosing to shame that person for how they've made us feel.

2. Storing moral credit

A lot of food trends that exist today have a focus on the health of the planet as well as the health of the person. These are based on the idea that certain ways of eating are better for the environment than others (whether this is true or not is another matter). In one interesting study on organic food, people were divided into three groups. The first were shown pictures of food labelled as organic, the second were shown pictures of typical comfort foods, and the third, the control group, were shown non-organic, non-comfort foods. All three groups were then asked to read brief descriptions of moral transgressions and were asked to judge these actions on a scale of one (not so bad) to seven (evil). They were also asked how much of their time they would be willing to volunteer to those in need. People who were shown the organic images were found to be more judgemental of the moral transgressions and less willing to volunteer their time. The theory behind this is that doing some-thing perceived as good for the planet like buying organic is seen as a way to store 'moral credit'. People feel like they've done their part, and this gives them the moral latitude to be super-judgemental about other people's behaviour and skimp on altruistic deeds. This is also a potential explanation for why militant vegans can sometimes be so cruel to other humans, because they feel they've done their bit for the animals, and this allows them some slack when it comes to humans. Obviously, it goes without saying that #NotAllVegans.

So we're quick to judge and shame others because we believe that the food choices someone makes tell us something funda-mental about them as a person, and because once we've done something seen as morally good (whether it's for ourselves or the planet) we feel (likely unconsciously) that allows us to be harsher to others. What makes these things so much more powerful on social media is the immediacy of it. We'll happily say things to people in the heat of the moment, including things we wouldn't say to someone if we encountered them on the street, because the screen barrier allows us some distance and a sense of anonymity. Plus, we feel a sense of entitlement to comment on someone's food choices because their profile is public.

3. Just world bias

Brené Brown, a research professor at the University of Houston, writes beautifully on shame, and shares in her work that we judge and shame others in areas where we ourselves feel vulnerable to shame. She writes: "We're hard on each other because we're using each other as a launching pad out of our own perceived shaming deficiency." If we're busy shaming others, it means the spotlight is not on us. If we shame others for the things we ourselves are most insecure about, that means that our food shaming likely stems from an uncertainty and sense of shame about our own eating, whether that's because we 'cheated' or because we're afraid of others perceiving us as 'lazy' or 'unmotivated'. Or maybe it's because we're afraid of being unwell.

We want to believe that if we just do the right things nothing bad will happen to us. On the flip side, we also therefore want to believe that if something bad happens to someone else that they have done something to deserve it. This is known as the 'just world bias', and explains a lot about the human tendency to victim blame. The idea is encapsulated in phrases like, 'they got what was coming' or 'what goes around comes around' – the idea that the world is inherently fair and just. Except it isn't. Good things and bad things often happen to those who don't deserve it. The most obvious example of just world bias in action is when we blame the victims of rape and assault, when we ask: 'what was she wearing?' or 'why did they drink alcohol?', and when we say 'you shouldn't have walked home alone in the dark'. We are far more comfortable latching onto something that person has done wrong, which must have led them to be assaulted, because if we know what they've done wrong we can avoid doing the wrong thing, and therefore avoid being assaulted ourselves. We think if we can avoid the behaviour of past victims, we won't be victims ourselves. Of course, it doesn't work like that; people are assaulted no matter what they wear and no matter how much they drink, and everyone has a right to be able to walk home without the fear of being attacked. The blame is firmly and totally with the attacker or rapist. In our rational minds we know this. But it scares us because it makes us vulnerable, and most of us have grown up believing vulnerability to be a weakness.

Applying this to social media, I've definitely been told by strangers, 'If you can't handle people's comments, you shouldn't be online', which is still a form of victim blaming. It implies it's my own fault I receive hurtful and abusive messages from people, because I'm a visible online figure. If that doesn't sound quite fair to you, it's because it's not. Yet we tell ourselves that if we don't do those things then we won't get nasty messages. (Spoiler alert: if you're a woman or gender non-conforming person on the Internet you will get nasty messages. It's unavoidable. If you're a person of any gender who stands up for what they believe in, people will try and take you down and revel in the process, because it makes them feel better about themselves. Just briefly though. It doesn't last.)

Alongside just world bias, our society has adopted a neoliberal model of healthism, which implies that health is purely the responsibility of the individual and health is a moral imperative for being a good person and a good citizen. Healthism neglects to consider all the factors outside of our individual control that can influence health: socioeconomic (income, education, employment, access to healthcare), environmental, genetic, accidents, and so on. It therefore implies that if you're unwell it's your own fault, because you're not making the right choices. When we have this pervasive message surrounding us, it invites us to shame each other for making the 'wrong' choices, as it firmly implies it *is* always a choice (it's really not). We do this because we are conditioned to by healthism, and because we are ourselves deeply afraid of making the 'wrong' choice.

Being critical of others' food choices is a way of externalising the criticism or self-control you apply to yourself. I strongly believe that people resort to food shaming and make cruel statements when they are jealous that you have a strong sense of self and a positive relationship with your body and food that they don't have. Some may be struggling with the restrictive set of rules they've given themselves but are so caught up in the morality and identity they've assigned to these rules that they can't easily let go. Others may just be in denial that the rules don't even really align with who they are.

Of course, it would be wrong to say that we always shame others from a place of insecurity. Sometimes we shame others because we're disappointed in their behaviour and want them to do better. We think this is an effective tool for behaviour change. It can be, but rarely, and often at the cost of that person's feelings of self-worth and self-esteem. We have decades of research that shows when we fat shame someone they are actually less likely to lose weight, and more likely to feel worse about themselves. It literally has the opposite effect to the one intended. It hurts rather than helps.

Other times, as in the case of Rawvana for example, we feel so angry and betrayed in that moment that we use the instant nature of social media to write something we either might regret or wouldn't have felt needed sharing had we taken some time away to process those emotions. I spoke to someone who used to follow Rawvana* who told me, "When I heard she was caught eating animal products earlier this year, my initial reaction was a 'serves you right' response. However, after hearing she had to abandon that lifestyle for health reasons, I was happy for her in a way. It's hard to build your entire brand and business around a certain lifestyle just to be told it's killing you, and I'm glad she now puts her health first. I only wish she had respectfully come clean about it instead of falsely selling the lifestyle. Not only was she faking it herself, but she knew the diet was causing health complications for her and was STILL selling it to people like us for profit."

You cannot eat anything or share a picture of any food these days without someone somewhere having an opinion on it, one they feel the need to share publicly to anyone who will listen.

---

* Who wanted to remain anonymous.

My eating is not my qualification

As a healthcare professional, I absolutely have felt the pressure to 'look healthy' and to model 'good' food choices in order to avoid shaming comments. It made me nervous whenever I posted food pictures online. Thankfully, I've worked past that and now couldn't give two shits what someone thinks about what I eat. But I'm far from the only one.

Zara, a dietetics student, shared a story about how one of her friends told her "I would've thought as a dietitian you'd know that's not healthy", despite the fact that everyone else was eating similar food to herself. She says, "It made me feel paranoid about what I eat and how people will view my future ability as a dietitian." These concerns aren't unfounded – there have been many instances where prominent voices on Twitter have stated that healthcare professionals shouldn't be trusted if they're not thin, as clearly that means they aren't able to follow their own advice. This is absolute rubbish. Someone's body size has no bearing on their professional qualifications. I have definitely received my fair share of comments like this on social media. But the key difference between my and Zara's experience is that I have a thinner body, whereas Zara is in a larger body.

"I started gaining weight in my early 20s and it was devastating to me," she shares. "I felt betrayed by my own body and didn't have an active social media presence. However, now that I'm a bit older, I tend to care about other people's opinions less. I do share a lot more with regards to my size... About two years ago I would only really show 'clean eating foods' whereas now I do show the homemade milkshakes and the tasty salads because there's got to be a balance."

I asked Zara if she stops herself from posting food pictures sometimes. She answered: "Not really, I want people to see what I eat. I personally can't stand feeds that are just an endless stream of salads, steamed food, and so on. I like a mix; I don't like being force-fed restrictions."

What Zara's story highlights is that the standards are different depending on how you look. If you're thin, you can be praised for eating a whole pizza with two pints of lager. Fat people, on the other hand, have to face strangers making strong inferences about them based on one meal or one item of food they eat. If they eat something 'healthy' they're told 'well clearly it isn't working', or 'nice try, we know you didn't eat that'. If they eat something 'unhealthy' they're told 'this is why you're fat and going to die of a heart attack at 30', or 'you're disgusting', or they are laughed at. (These are all genuine comments people have told me they've received online.)

Clearly we all know that one doughnut or one salad doesn't mean anything in the grand scheme of things, and doesn't have that much power, but we so easily assume that the salad must be an anomaly and the doughnut must be a regular occurrence, because our assumption is based on appearance. It's important to say that, regardless of whether these assumptions are right or wrong, it absolutely does not give anyone the right to say such horrible things online. All people are deserving of basic human respect, no matter their appearance.

Food shaming is a weighty issue

Fat people are far more likely to be shamed for their food choices, both online and in person. In addition, anyone speaking about a health condition online can expect to receive unsolicited advice on a regular basis and receive shaming comments about either ignoring or declining said advice. Michelle Elman is one of my favourite people on social media. She is incredible: a body confidence coach, body positive activist and all-round wonderful human. She says: "I don't think it's helpful or healthy to share the food you eat online because no matter what you share, it is taking someone's diet out of context by usually only sharing one or two meals a day. For the influencer, I think it's a lot of pressure to eat healthier to not receive abuse and it comes with a message of 'if you eat how I eat, you will look like me'. If you are a fat influencer, then it opens you up to comments like 'no wonder you are the size that you are'." Michelle has received her fair share of disbelieving comments on her eating because of her body. "I have shared a few 'what I eat in a day' videos in the past on YouTube and whilst it isn't content I would create today, at the time, I got a lot of 'I'm shocked you eat so healthy', 'I don't believe this is what you eat at your size', 'you can't be this size and be vegetarian' (I'm not vegetarian but I don't eat a lot of meat and can enjoy a meal with or without meat just as much)."

Sasha (see pages 108 110), who has Crohn's disease, fell into the 'clean eating' movement to regain a sense of control over her eating. She says seeing these shiny happy 'cured' people on social media talking about their eating habits made her feel ashamed, and "seeing clean eating credited as the source of this recovery almost made me feel like I wasn't trying hard enough to 'cure' myself if I didn't start following a diet that could be described as clean eating". So she started eating 'clean' and, at first, she felt empowered and in control. "Then, I gradually became more anxious of eating the 'wrong' food or of having to go out for a meal and there not being a vegan option. Or 'contaminating' my body with gluten or dairy. The whole subject of food and eating became the sole focus of my life so, in that sense, had a detrimental effect to my wellbeing, even if I didn't realise it at the time. Only with hindsight can I see that I was really unhappy."

Sasha still struggles with food to this day and avoids posting publicly about her condition to avoid unsolicited advice and shaming comments that she's seen others receive online. Others like Becky Excell.

Becky is a blogger and content creator who suffers from IBS and has to avoid gluten to manage her symptoms. When I asked her if she received unsolicited advice, her answer was a resounding: "Yes, a lot! With my gut health problems (IBS) I get people messaging me on a daily basis giving advice. I do find that some people can be very insistent and demanding in their advice, especially when they continue to see I'm struggling with my stomach (which I document on my Instagram Stories from time to time). I often get people messaging me telling me to try certain medication; I get people who have never met me trying to diagnose my issues and telling me what I should do. And don't get me started on the amount of people who advise me that a food intolerance test would be a good idea. To be honest I just ignore all of this advice. I know who I should and shouldn't listen to. I know many people do give advice with the best intentions online, but good intentions aren't enough."

Food shaming is a beauty issue

Another condition that seems to particularly attract unsolicited advice and shaming comments is acne. Dr Anjali Mahto is a consultant dermatologist who not only helps her patients manage their acne, but has struggled with persistent adult acne herself. On her Instagram account she documented a message she received from a follower that read: "No wonder you get such terrible acne. So much sugar and dairy all the time. Cocktails, ice cream...oil. Ugh. Prescribing is the easy route but at the end of the day laziness around lifestyle choices just won't help, no matter what any dermatologist says."

Anjali says she felt "indignant surprise" when she first received this message, then decided to use it to spread an important message. She wrote: "Commenting and giving people uninvited advice about their skin in such a negative manner is unnecessary, unkind and hurtful. For those people who are already struggling with how they look, messages like this aren't simply rude but actually nasty and can have deep, long-lasting effects on their mental health. The use of language in the message isn't to be ignored – words such as 'terrible' and 'ugh' and 'laziness' convey emotions of disgust and judgement. Blame is being applied to the sufferer that somehow their 'terrible' skin problem is because of their own 'laziness'. This is not OK. Acne is a medical problem, largely down to hormones and genetics – it is not a lifestyle one caused by ice cream on a hot day. Blaming and judging people for their skin disease or dietary choices is unacceptable from a social interaction point of view and simply wrong from a scientific one." I think she hits the nail on the head there.

P is a genderqueer human who has experienced severe cystic acne. They said they had mild acne for a good ten years until it "exploded out of nowhere" with no identifiable cause in 2018. The only thing that's worked for them is isotretinoin (branded as Roaccutane or Accutane) – a drug that has been subjected to a lot of fearmongering online, but which is undeniably effective and safe in the right hands.

They tried some diet adjustments while their acne was still mild. "I cut out dairy a few times, I was vegan for probably about 2 years, and I tried to convince myself it was for ethical reasons, but in reality, it was always to do with my skin. All of these things had come from reading about it and hearing other people talking about it online. If you Google 'acne' very quickly you will find 'top diets for acne' and I had in my head for all these years that my skin is like this because I haven't cracked the right diet yet or made the right choices."

"Because of the emphasis on diet, anyone who's known skin problems has this idea of 'I did this to myself', 'I caused this'. It's a huge source of shame for a lot of people, including me, I always felt like I deserved this because I had been lazy, not eaten the right foods, couldn't fix it, and so on. So on top of the insecurities about the way you look you also feel like you only have yourself to blame."

These feelings of shame (to which social media absolutely contributes) meant P was reluctant to go to a doctor because they felt not only that it wasn't serious enough, but also that they had done this to themselves. P did eventually consult a dermatologist and has absolutely no regrets about it. "I asked my dermatologist if I could have done this to myself, and the doctor said absolutely not. It was such a relief!"

Acne often carries a huge amount of self-blame with it, likely because of the way it crosses over into the realm of beauty and aesthetics, and so people with acne can be accused of being vain. Having acne doesn't match the standard of beauty we have in society of perfect flawless skin, and the idea of glowing skin being a marker of health. On top of that, you see a huge number of messages online from people who claim that acne is a symptom of a bad diet, which P has first-hand experience of. P posts about their skin on Instagram, which has attracted regular comments from strangers, "In the earlier days when my skin was at its worst it was a common occurrence for people to comment 'clean up your diet' or 'fix your diet'." These comments are vague, and don't actually offer any useful solutions at all, not to mention the audacity to assume that someone's diet *must* be bad because of their physical appearance (I've definitely heard that somewhere before...). P would sometimes receive more specific advice like 'cut out dairy', but on the whole it was a vague assumption that they were eating wrong.

"I have had a few people who follow the Medical Medium – I wasn't really aware of him – who were telling me I have to fix my body from the inside out, and that modern medicine just covers up problems and it's going to come back, so it's my fault for not addressing the real problem. It's clever how they use shame to try and convert you to celery juice." Clever and yet also exceptionally arrogant and patronising.

I've already discussed some theories as to why people food shame, but I was keen to hear what P thought: "I think they like to think that they're helping, but it's more that they want to feel heard and want to justify those decisions for themselves. They think 'I've given up dairy so I'm going to make someone else do it too', which I find quite strange." These kinds of comments are common within the acne community as well, where people will vocalise how they could have taken medication but have chosen not to as they want to 'heal naturally'.

So, how do they respond to these shaming comments and unsolicited advice? "It depends on what kind of day I'm having. I often just delete these comments now. Anyone who's coming from a place of needing to be heard is not going to listen, they're not doing it to have a conversation, they're simply doing it to get it out of their system. There's absolutely no point a lot of the time in trying to turn it into a two-way conversation, so I just delete the comments."

P adds, "I'm also keen to delete advice comments because I don't want others to see them. I've read through popular comment threads under acne posts and felt so much worse about myself, so I don't want to leave anything on my posts that could be harmful to people."

Interestingly, P receives more patronising comments from women, who are more likely to misgender them as male. Tied in with this whole narrative of 'healing naturally' is the idea that P's body is wrong because they are genderqueer. "When people are trying to find out the cause of my acne (and they're far more interested in a cause than I am!) hormones often comes up as people think I'm taking testosterone, because people's understanding of transgender presentation is very binary, and that everyone who is trans has to be on a path of some kind that makes sense to them. It's very accusatory." This again contributes to the narrative of blame, that someone has 'done this to themselves' by taking hormones, which, yes, can contribute to the development of acne in some trans folk, but doesn't make it OK to tell someone that they're 'messing up their body'.

P has accepted that their acne has no clear identifiable cause, and while other people's interest amuses them, to me it very much speaks to the just world bias mentioned earlier. People want to reduce their chances of experiencing acne, so they want to know what they can do to ensure they won't, by finding out what caused it in others.

One of the things that keeps P on Instagram is the part of the acne community that is supportive. Seeing your skin represented in a way that you just don't see in the media, hearing other people voice thoughts you've had for a while, seeing everyday people just being themselves and not hiding their acne, and hearing other people talking about food in a balanced, helpful, non-shaming way.

Food shaming is pervasive, and has more recently manifested itself in the form of environmentalism and sustainability, where eco bloggers are held to impossible standards and called hypocritical if they so much as eat chicken once, jump on an aeroplane to fly to another country, or have a drink that came with a plastic straw they didn't ask for. There are so many more examples I could offer, but hopefully the picture is clear: this is a widespread issue.

How can we counter food shaming?

Shaming comments can have a lot of power over how we feel about ourselves. As humans, we tend to give far more weight to negatives than positives. You could receive a hundred positive comments, but the one nasty shaming one will stay with you. You end up giving far more mental energy to the negative comments. Here are some examples of how you could reply.

WHAT THEY SAY	HOW TO REPLY
'Are you going to eat THAT?'	'Yes, I am!' (with confidence)
'I thought you're eating healthy?'	'Health is more complex than one food'
'I bet you didn't really eat that'	'Why would I post a picture of food I haven't eaten? I did eat it, and it was delicious'
'That looks gross'	'It tastes amazing – surely that's the most important thing?!'
'You need to improve your diet'	'You need to improve your manners. Please stop making assumptions about my eating'
'Diabetes in a cup/bowl'	'Fuck off' (to be honest this works as a response to most things)
[Insert pretty much any shaming comment here]	[Instant and loud changing of the subject to something far more interesting]

It can be helpful to remind ourselves that people who write hateful and shaming comments are generally not coming from a happy place, and that they tend to be quite insecure about themselves. They are putting you down to make themselves feel bigger. Knowing that can make a huge difference, that and asking yourself 'why do I value this person's opinion?'

As someone who has been on social media since 2012, I have received so many horrible comments online. To a certain extent, you develop a thicker skin after a while, and these comments usually don't get to me in quite the same way they used to. I have no desire to romanticise my resilience here, as I shouldn't have had to develop it in the first place.

We admire the kind of tenacity that comes with having a thick skin, even though behind the scenes there are usually consequences. I may not be reduced to tears any more by the comments I receive, but they still hurt, and if I receive too many I know I need to step away, turn off comments, reach out to friends, remind myself that I'm good at my job, and do things I know will make me happy. In particular, as a recovering perfectionist, it can get right to the heart of my insecurities when people shame me for making mistakes.

Speaking of perfectionism, the whole idea of a 'perfect diet' needs to be discussed.

5

AM I EATING PERFECTLY?

Stating that social media helps spread misinformation is not exactly news to most people. Mention this to a group of people and you're more likely to hear 'duh, of course' rather than 'what, really?!' in response. We're all aware that social media is one of the biggest sources of information, and therefore misinformation, out there, and yet we continue to fall for it.

Social media is contributing to a significant level of food anxiety in people, in terms of specific foods, and also in terms of the general pressure to eat well, or even 'perfectly'.

Are you anxious about what to eat?

Most people who walk through the door into my clinic room come because they have a relationship with food that is riddled with fear, shame and anxiety. They have been exposed to a significant amount of misinformation (usually online) and they're tired of feeling stressed about everything they're eating. They want greater freedom with food.

Anxiety is part of the body's stress response, also known as 'fight or flight'. When this is triggered, it causes adrenaline and cortisol to be released in the body, which has a number of effects, including raised heart rate and blood pressure, and quicker breathing, with blood rushing to your muscles in case you need to use them to get away. The fight or flight response is incredibly useful in dangerous situations, but it can also be triggered by perfectly safe foods due to a fear that the food will cause harm.

There are a number of reasons, but the one I see most often is that someone has read about how this food will cause cancer, diabetes, weight gain, acne or any other condition, or an overall worry that this food is 'bad' for them in some way.

To work through the length and breadth of health and nutrition misinformation online would be a whole book in itself.* The democratisation of social media, and the fact that we all eat, has made everyone a self-appointed expert in food. The side effect of this is people following the advice of well-meaning influencers with a severe case of Dunning-Kruger.†

When I have a discussion with someone in clinic, I often ask them to make a list of their food anxieties, and from there we

---

* You'll find some of the common foods that are sources of anxiety for people, as well as a discussion of why people fall for misinformation, in my first book, *The Wellness Rebel*.

† The Dunning-Kruger effect is a cognitive bias whereby people have an inability to recognise their incompetence. They know a little about something, and yet have no idea just how much they don't know. The effect can also be summarised by the phrase 'a little knowledge is a dangerous thing'. Generally, the more of an expert you are in something, the more you realise how much you still have to learn.

talk about where these ideas may have come from. Sometimes individuals point to a terrible propaganda piece – sorry, 'documentary' – on Netflix. Sometimes it's an elusive 'I've seen it in so many places', and other times they will be able to name a specific post by a specific person on social media.

The origin of these food anxieties matters, as a fear that came from social media is very different from a fear that originated from legitimate medical advice. It can also help people identify if there's a clear pattern of origins, which might be just the wake-up call they need to reassess their relationship with social media in general, and let go of the idea of there being a perfect way of eating they need to emulate.

Are you eating the perfect diet?

Anyone who has any kind of audience online can feel that pressure to model the perfect diet. It's very much linked to the issue of food shaming, as we think if we have the perfect diet then no one can shame or judge us for what we're eating. But, of course, that isn't the case, because what is a 'perfect' or even a 'good' diet seems to be incredibly subjective, online as well as offline.

From a scientific perspective, there's no such thing as the perfect diet. Those who preach a one-size-fits-all approach are quacks who generally want to sell you a diet plan, or zealots who are so invested in the way they're eating that they can't imagine why anyone else would want to eat differently. There is no ideal diet for everyone. There will be a pattern of eating that is more suited to a particular individual, but the reasons behind that are incredibly complex (genetics, culture, medical conditions, upbringing, likes and dislikes, etc.), and this pattern will very likely not be the same for you as the person next to you.

Cassidy is a nutrition student, who avoids posting about the food she eats online because of the pressure to model a 'perfect' diet. "I feel as someone that studies nutrition I am expected to always be eating some beautiful salad or smoothie that I have made. Often my flatmates would tease me about eating relatively the same boring meals all the time or question my lack of eating that resulted from the constant teasing. Even to the point, one flatmate mentioned to their personal tutor that I wasn't one to go to for meal ideas. It seems if you study nutrition you are either assumed to be vegan or constantly eating a wide array of different meals that contain only fruit and vegetables."

Whether you have a large platform, are in a position of authority, or simply know that all your friends are watching your social media accounts, it can add a huge pressure to be 'perfect'.

Now, don't get me wrong, if social media was driving people to make healthier food choices then I'd be totally here for that; I'm a nutritionist after all! Sometimes, this is the case for someone. What I often see instead, however, is a pressure to make the 'right' decision that ends up leaving people with worse mental health issues than before, and a restrictive diet based on misinformation that isn't as balanced or varied as it could be.

In fact, there is evidence to suggest that the more you look at perfectly positioned and captured food images, the less likely you are to make that food. In other words, making food pictures look *too* perfect actually discourages people from making the dish. This is the opposite of what we've been led to believe, as we want to post pictures of delicious-looking food to entice customers. If the photographed food is something people can buy, then it's not an issue, perfection sells. But when it comes to cooking food ourselves – which is what a lot of bloggers are trying to help people to do – the picture has to seem realistic and achievable enough for your average person to want to give it a go. Overly beautiful staged photos can be intimidating or seem unrealistic, like a fantasy food rather than something tangible they can reproduce.

Generation perfect

The millennial generation has been labelled the 'perfectionist generation'. Research shows that the majority of millennials are experiencing multidimensional perfectionism – a pressure to meet increasingly high standards – as measured by a set of metrics. This perfectionism has been linked to a growing number of cases of mental illness in millennials, including eating disorders, anxiety and depression. Perfectionism is making us ill.

Perfectionism is often seen as a strength disguised as a weakness. When you're asked in an interview "What's your greatest weakness?", declaring that you're a perfectionist is a safe answer. Perfectionism is also often mistaken for 'being perfect' or 'doing something perfectly', and therefore people assume that it must be a good thing. It can be; perfectionism can allow us to have ambition, aim high, and achieve incredible things. This is more generally known as adaptive perfectionism, and it's adaptive because it motivates people to do well and to have ambition without being paralysed by a fear of failure. Adaptive perfectionists derive a sense of pleasure from working hard at something, but also allow themselves some flexibility. Any successes that person achieves boosts their self-esteem, so they take pride in their skills, and acknowledge their achievement. Alongside this, they are able to take their own limitations and strengths into account. In this way, adaptive perfectionism is flexible and helpful.

Maladaptive perfectionists, on the other hand, never seem to be satisfied even when they do their best, as there is always something they feel they could have done better. 'Good enough' is never good enough. This form of perfectionism involves putting pressure on themselves to meet high standards which then powerfully influence the way that person thinks about themselves. They judge their self-worth based on their ability to strive for and achieve unrelentingly high standards.

Although having high standards is generally a good thing, perfectionists are doomed to failure, because they set themselves standards that are simply not attainable for humans. It's the equivalent of needing to get 100% in everything, even if 80% is a grade 'A' and no one else will ever know the difference. This puts someone in a vulnerable position, as not reaching these insanely high standards feels like a personal failure, even if by objective standards it was good enough, and can have a significantly detrimental impact on someone's health and wellbeing.

The thought patterns behind maladaptive perfectionism are typically all-or-nothing thinking ('If I don't get an A I've failed'), using 'should' and 'must' ('I *should* be able to do this easily'), and fear of failure ('If I don't do well others will think I'm useless'). Underlying these are assumptions about ourselves, for example, 'If I don't do my job perfectly then I will get fired' or 'If I'm not the perfect partner they will leave me', or 'If I don't succeed then I'm a worthless person'. These assumptions tend to be rigid and inaccurate, making them particularly unhelpful.

Some people seem to be perfectionists from birth, whereas others learn to become perfectionists from their environment; from parents, school, friends, partners or social media. You can test yourself in the final chapter with the Multidimensional Perfectionism Scale* – the most commonly used tool for assessing perfectionism. The original scale includes six categories: concern over mistakes, doubts about actions, personal standards, organisation, parental criticism and parental expectations. Concern over mistakes involves a preoccupation with mistakes to such an extent that performance is either perfect or worthless, success or failure. Doubts about actions characterise a nagging sense of doubt regarding how well something has been executed. Personal standards reflect setting unreasonably high personal standards and goals. Organisation includes an overemphasis on order, precision and neatness. Parental criticism and parental expectations involve perceptions of parents as being overly critical and holding unrealistically high expectations. Not every perfectionist will score highly in every one of those categories.

Do others think you're perfect?

While perfectionism manifests as a desire to *be* perfect, it can also appear as the desire to *look* perfect. This desire to be perceived as perfect by others in order to gain approval is referred to as 'socially prescribed perfectionism'. It is a need to publicly portray

---

* There is a version of this scale that includes three different sections: other-oriented perfectionism, self-oriented perfectionism and socially prescribed perfectionism. However, I'm assuming you, the reader, will be most interested in the last two, so the quiz will focus on those.

a flawless image to others and involves regular self-monitoring and manipulation of behaviour to fit with each situation. The appearance of perfection is far more important here than reality.

While all forms of perfectionism have increased in the past three decades, socially prescribed perfectionism has risen the most – by 33% – between 1989 and 2016. Why is this? Of course, it's easy to blame social media, but there's more to it than that. Although we millennials didn't necessarily grow up with social media in our childhood, we did have it throughout our teens and/or adulthood, and this has had a significant effect on our wellbeing.

We have cultivated a modern landscape that says the perfect life and perfect lifestyle exist. We've also pushed the narrative that nothing is out of reach if we only try hard enough. In essence: the perfect life and perfect lifestyle are available to anyone, provided you try hard enough. But that's not true, this meritocracy is an illusion. We've been taught from an early age to define ourselves by numbers – exam scores, percentiles, league tables – and social media preys on that by attaching a number to our popularity: likes, follows, comments and shares.

Anyone with an Instagram account can probably relate to this. We're now being encouraged to think of our public life as a performance rather than something we participate in. We feel the need to measure up to our peers, which is easily examined given that we have so much access to other people's celebrations, achievements, holidays and lifestyle. We crave validation, and we can judge others almost as harshly as we judge ourselves.

From a young age we have been taught that metrics and rankings matter. Our grades were constantly compared to others, our schools and universities ranked in league tables, all part of a constant comparison. When Facebook launched, initially it was available only to students – truly the perfect customers, desperate for the validation it offered. When we go online, we're surrounded by platforms that appear to be full of other people meeting these goals. Intellectually, we know it's all a highlight reel, but emotionally it's a struggle. Social media has created a world where everyone's achievements are on public display, amplifying our need to live up to a societal model of perfection. Yet another space where we can set ourselves impossibly high standards; yet another space in which to fear failure. It sounds exhausting.

Social media amplifies perfectionistic tendencies like a megaphone, taking our personal lives and making them publicly available for scrutiny, so that these aspects of our lives become another stick with which to beat ourselves when we fall short, or yet another way to seek validation from others that we're doing the right thing. Even by using hearts as its primary metric, Instagram enables people to conflate attention with affection.

We've already discussed the concept of using food as a way to control how we are perceived by others in chapter 1, as we make assumptions about each other based on what we consume. I believe this perfectionism is a specific and particularly harmful example of this image presentation, which is partly fuelled by comparison. People are posting their best pictures and their best selves online, so of course when you compare your mundane everyday life to this highlight reel you fall short and feel as if you're not good enough. Add perfectionism to this and the pressure to post the 'perfect' picture to portray the 'perfect' life becomes even greater. But this is an impossible goal, as there will always be someone who has (or at least appears to have) a more perfect life than yours, and social media makes those people especially easy to find.

Some young people now have both a public Instagram page that portrays a 'perfect' life, and another 'fake' Instagram account, known as a 'finsta', where they post with less pressure, are less worried about being judged, share opinions and have more open discussions. For example, they may post a picture of their family holiday on their 'main' Instagram and post their weekend underage drinking with friends on the 'finsta' page to avoid being judged. Others call it a 'shinsta' – a 'shit Instagram'* page where they can post their failures and make fun of them, again without judgement. Their perceived flaws are available for only their closest friends to see. Interestingly, some students are fully conscious and aware that they are using Instagram for this exact purpose, and yet you may wonder why they don't just delete the 'main' Instagram page? It's because it's seen as a networking tool and to be seen by others to be active online.

One of the big issues with social media perfectionism is that more and more young people are joining sites like Instagram and are exposed to this content from a younger age. Having more perfectionistic influences and triggers early on can lead to a greater risk of harm: as perfectionists grow older, the harmful aspects of perfectionism can develop unchecked. Perfectionists become more prone to anxiety, guilt and envy, and actually become less organised and disciplined, as the fear of failure reaches a point where it's crippling. In fact, pursuing the fleeting goal of perfection can result in a higher rate of failure over time.

---

*   I spoke to some of my younger Gen Z clients, and several of them confirmed that this is, in fact, a real thing.

Overall, then, our results suggest life does not get easier for perfectionists. In a challenging, messy and imperfect world, perfectionists may burn out as they age, leaving them more unstable and less able to cope.

Buying perfection

Hilariously, there is now a way to give the impression online that you're living your best life without having to make any effort whatsoever. In 2018 a new start-up appeared called LifeFaker.com, which claimed to be 'the world's first online life faking service'. It is a website where users can buy ready-to-post photo packages they can pass off as their own. Its mission statement encapsulates this madness exquisitely: 'Life isn't perfect. Your profile should be. Instead of going to the trouble of living a perfect life, now you can just get the photos instead.'

LifeFaker's photo packages are every Instagram stereotype you could imagine. These include the 'Look At My Holiday and Cry Package', the 'I Found Love and Babies Package', the 'My Weekend Was Amazing Thanks Package', and the 'Look What I Had for Lunch Package'.

If right now you're rolling your eyes and despairing, then I have good news for you, because the company isn't quite what it seems. Anyone who tries to buy a package will be redirected to Sanctus, the start-up behind the initiative. The site reminds us that we've all felt the pressures of social media and invites us to watch a film that explores how unhealthy behaviours on social media affect us and what we can do to change them.

Perfectionism + Social Media = Orthorexia

Social media is a perfectionist's dream and nightmare: when perfectionism meets social media, it's a dangerous self-perpetuating cycle. In the context of food, social media becomes the vehicle to 'perform' perfect eating to gain the validation and praise needed to reassure us that we're doing the right thing.

In some cases, food perfectionism and food anxiety morph into a condition termed orthorexia, particularly as maladaptive perfectionists are at higher risk of developing this disorder. While orthorexia usually begins as a desire to overcome illness or improve health, it becomes obsessive, with a fixation on the purity and 'perfect' nutritional value of food. This becomes a focus on physical health at the expense of mental health and social interactions, and, in severe cases, can lead to malnutrition and vitamin deficiencies. Although the focus is very much on health, in practice it is almost impossible to separate health and thinness, as society sees them as equal and the same. Orthorexia is more socially acceptable than other kinds of eating disorder because it cultivates, or rather, it performs healthy behaviours, and usually includes thinness as part of the package. This makes orthorexia difficult to spot.

Researchers have also added to this definition of orthorexia, extending it to a behavioural disorder rooted in a deeper social pathology, such as perfectionism, desire to conform, feelings of moral superiority, and a strong desire to control health status.

The most famous case of orthorexia is the blogger Jordan Younger, formerly known as the Blonde Vegan to her social media followers. Younger's orthorexic behaviour began with a desire to improve her health, as she claims she has always struggled with her gut health and various digestive issues. She became vegan, started going on juice cleanses that she said made her feel great, and began sharing her 'health journey' on her blog and Instagram. Her following grew and she became so successful she was making a living producing sponsored content and selling items such as yoga gear and cleanses on her website. Her memoir, *Breaking Vegan*, tells the story of how her eating became more and more restrictive, more and more obsessive, and more and more anxiety-inducing for her, all laid bare on social media for people to see and imitate. She rebranded from the Blonde Vegan into the Balanced Blonde. In her memoir she reveals that behind the smiling Instagram facade she was consumed with guilt over her food choices, anxiety over her health, and was unable to enjoy spending time with family or friends unless she had complete control over what she could eat. Her eating became more and more extreme, to the point where there was only one green juice from a specific cafe that she felt comfortable eating when out and about. At her breaking point, she ate some salmon and never looked back. Younger describes the moment where she revealed to her followers that she was no longer vegan as being terrifying, and she received significant backlash for turning her back on veganism. She says she lost a lot of followers, and even received death threats. However, the good news for her was that she gained significant media attention and a book deal. She still blogs, posts on her Instagram, has a podcast, and seems really into yoga. You get the feeling she is on a continual quest to improve herself – or, rather, her body – and never seems satisfied. She may claim that she has moved on from her orthorexia, but a quick scroll through her social media accounts suggests otherwise. While she may no longer be living off green juices, she is promoting water fasting, parasite detox protocols, and all manner of quack treatments in her pursuit of wellness. From an outside perspective, it is clear that her obsession with health is still very much intact, and that her orthorexia has likely just shifted focus.

Orthorexia is a disorder of excess but also of confusion in the face of excess. Excess in terms of food abundance, but also in terms of the health information that exists online.

Chartered psychologist Kimberley Wilson says: "I work with a range of psychological issues (not all food-related) but social media has been a perpetuating factor for everyone I have worked with who has had a restrictive eating disorder – anorexia, orthorexia, food anxiety. In these cases, clients describe how information they read on social media maintains their anxieties about reintroducing 'unsafe' foods, or how 'fitspo'-type images undermine their body esteem/autonomy. It may be that clients dealing with bulimia and compulsive eating issues also have a harmful relationship with social media but that it is less prominent with these kinds of issues."

Are you the perfect parent?

One group of people in particular who are particularly vulnerable to messages of perfectionism online are parents: particularly when pregnant, breastfeeding and weaning.

Becoming a parent is arguably one of the most stressful life events a human can go through and represents a time when new mothers are at increased risk of developing mood and anxiety disorders. Maternal wellbeing has also been linked with perfectionism, as mothers with perfectionistic tendencies have been shown in research to display poorer parental adjustment, increased anxiety, and lowered self-efficacy. Socially prescribed parenting perfectionism involves the belief that society holds high standards for their parenting, something which is heavily exacerbated by social media.

Recently, a new generation of mummy bloggers have been born: fitness and wellness bloggers who have a baby and start sharing their advice interwoven with their personal story. Their pregnancies are portrayed as glowing celebrations of woman-hood while their husbands lovingly kiss their bellies at every opportunity. (Oh, the heteronormativity of it all!) Any mention of morning sickness is accompanied by a smoothie recipe with 500 ingredients you can only find at organic health shops and looks like it would induce sickness, not cure it. The story of birth is paired with smiling images with no mention of pain whatsoever. The baby food is all homemade in their #gifted blender because god forbid you're too tired to give your child the 'perfect' 'natural' food. All in all, pregnancy and motherhood are simply a shiny happy extension of their shiny perfect, pain-free lives. It's 'positive vibes only' to the point where it's not simply unrealistic but can cause harm to others.

Given the link between perfectionism and poor maternal mental health, social media platforms may present as a particular risk factor for mothers who strive for perfection and compare themselves to the ideals presented on social media. In fact, in a UK survey in 2017 more than 80% of women said that Instagram and Facebook 'added pressure to be the perfect mum'. When people are comparing themselves to these privileged idealised images of parenting, they may feel that they're not having a good enough pregnancy, that they're not looking after their baby as well as they could. Plus, they often reinforce traditional gender stereotypes and unequal gender roles, which may contribute to parenting stress in mothers. There is a heavy focus on being 'perfectly imperfect' – perfect hair and make-up but, oops, a few toys on the floor! These 'perfectly imperfect' mums aren't helping women transition into motherhood. In fact, they may be more harmful than the ones who peddle perfection. As Nadine Cheung wrote for the magazine *VICE*: "Perfectly imperfect content is a way to commiserate with women on a superficial level without revealing any wounds that are deeper than a paper cut. This can lead to more feelings of isolation and deter new moms from seeking help from a professional when they need it the most."

Underlying this is an incredible stigma surrounding any negative comments about pregnancy and parenting, for fear of being called a bad parent, particularly for the person giving birth to and breastfeeding (or not) the baby. Given this, I do think it is understandable that people are afraid of being publicly shamed, and so hide anything that could be perceived as negative about the whole experience. But that doesn't negate the fact that this is simply perpetuating the cycle of perfectionism, fear and shame.

I'm by no means an expert on parenting, but thankfully Charlotte Stirling-Reed is. Charlotte is a registered nutritionist and expert in maternal and infant nutrition, and she also happens to have given birth to a beautiful boy, Raffy.

Charlotte agrees that social media can add an extra pressure for expectant mothers to have the 'perfect' pregnancy. "There are a lot of pages which do show more of the positive 'glowing' sides to pregnancy as well as advice pages that can essentially put a lot of pressure on expectant mums. The problem that often comes as a result of social media, seems to be comparison. Comparing your own pregnancy journey with someone else's is never going to be helpful, especially when the person on the other side of the screen has a completely different life, including genetics, family histories, likes and dislikes and environments. On the other hand, there are a growing number of IG accounts who really try to show the 'realities' of pregnancy, parenting and everything in-between. I think the public are craving honesty to help normalise some of the difficulties that many parents and pregnant women may face during their journeys."

Charlotte posts about her own experience being a mother to Raffy on her social media, using a combination of her personal story and the evidence base. "As with everything we talk about in nutrition, there has to be some balance, but first, parents need confidence! That's my main aim in the work I do, to provide information to give parents the confidence to feed their children well. Once they have that confidence it can make everything else easier."

Because of this, she receives a large number of comments and questions online on a daily basis. "I think lots of pregnant women have all the intentions in the world to exercise, eat healthily and take care of themselves, but the realities are often so far from the picture that they've painted. This is because life/ symptoms often get in the way. I guess parents often want or ask for some 'quick fix' advice to help them eat well or stay healthy or even to reduce the symptoms they might be feeling during pregnancy. Often there isn't a quick-fix solution, and, for some, healthy eating and exercise might also be completely out of the question. Everyone's pregnancy is just so unique, so you'll never know before how each of them will turn out. You can only try to remember you're human and do your best as well as make sure you take care of yourself and put yourself first, for once."

Charlotte also has some strong views about a lot of these mummy forums on the Internet: "My thoughts are also that some of the online forums really don't help with parental anxiety. There is a lot of misinformation, sure, but there is also a lot of judgement between and towards parents, as well as lots of black and white thinking about HOW we should feed children. Again, children (and families) are unique and science/feeding/nutrition is NEVER black and white. There is no right and wrong, just balance and realism."

So what effect does she think this is having on the health of the mother? "The pressure to do it all and to be everything to everyone is REAL as a parent. I definitely feel it in my work/life/parenting experiences too. It's hard when you look at social media every day and see everyone getting on with life, exercising every day, eating beautiful bowls of salads, being successful in their work. It's SO hard not to notice this and compare, especially on a hard day. Parents often have to juggle. A lot. It's a hard job as it is, and I think the comparisons with others who have seemingly 'nailed it' make us feel pretty worthless sometimes. You have to remind yourself that a) social media isn't reality, b) what's right for you isn't what's right for another mother and family, and c) YOU are enough."

Status

According to Kimberley Wilson, it's not all just about perfectionism, it's also about status. "We are compelled to try to elevate our social standing in relation to our peers. On some parts of social media that means posing on the bonnets of supercars with handfuls of cash and expensive handbags. On others it is about going on stylish holidays. And for some it is about having the 'best' body whether that is achieved through physical transformation or rarefied food choices. So, thinking psychologically, I would say it is less about 'having it all' and more of an anxious defence against being found wanting or judged as inadequate in some way."

This is very true. Status is based on beliefs about who the members of a society believe holds comparatively more or less social value. When it comes to social media, we have started to equate likes and followers with an elevated social status. There are unspoken rules online, for example tactically posting at certain times of day when your followers are more likely to be online, all for the purpose of getting as many likes as possible. Some people I know are afraid to post pictures of themselves rather than food because they get so few likes and several unfollows. We do not want to appear insignificant. More likes, more follows and more friends all equate to more public recognition that you have an interesting, active life.

Each social media platform has a hierarchy: those people who have high status have to stay active in order to maintain that status – not posting would mean slipping – and those who don't have status keep posting in order to try and become someone who has status. In reality, almost everyone on social media is constantly trying to climb higher and higher, but this social hierarchy reinforces models of perfection, constantly keeping us in a state of status anxiety, making us feel deficient in some way. Somebody is always ahead of us in some respect, whether it's more followers or a life that's closer to what we want, which inevitably leads to comparison, and that keeps us feeling like we need to post more in order to keep up and measure up: when you post on Facebook it's literally called a *status* update.

This is why Instagram food porn works: it transforms an indulgent meal or snack from a physical activity into a status performance. In the most successful trends, posting a picture of a particular food item signals social status in the form of affluence and being 'in the know'. When someone has to queue for hours in line for a cronut, or finds the best freakshake laden with an entire week's worth of chocolate and sweets, it signals that not only can you afford to spend your money on something so clearly ridiculous yet popular, you can also afford to spend hours waiting for it and photographing it. This idea is captured in the popular phrase: 'pics, or it didn't happen.'

The most notable part of these kinds of food photos is that something is clearly missing: the actual eating of the food. Instead, the item is displayed as some kind of trophy. Instagram food has almost nothing to do with consumption as a gastronomic exercise. Instead, consuming Instagrammable food means acquiring it, and sharing proof of your achievement. This reduces it from a sensory experience into an aesthetic one.

Deliberate imperfection

As always, where there is a movement on social media, there is a countermovement, and corners of the Internet exist that are actively countering the culture of food perfectionism online in the most beautifully imperfect ways. Enter: Dimly Lit Meals for One on Tumblr. Described as 'heartbreaking tales of sad food and even sadder lives', it pairs grainy photos of barely plated culinary monstrosities with a fictional tale about the sad lonely person who is likely eating it. The photos are submitted by real people, who often include a brief description of what the food in the image is. This, it turns out, is kind of important, as it's often difficult to tell by sight. Take a look at some of the contributions and you'll see what I mean. Since this project's humble beginnings on Tumblr in 2014, it has become such a success that you can now buy the published book.

These meals are the polar opposite of what you'll find on popular Instagram accounts: foods eaten straight out of cans, beige on beige, all harsh shadows and unappealing textures. Think bread rolls stuffed with salami, crisp sandwiches, mashed potato with an unidentifiable meat in gravy so watery it looks like piss, and a plate of pasta with an upended can of tuna on top.

Also on Tumblr, we have Sad Desk Lunch, showcasing tragic al-desko meals from overworked employees with the tagline: '62% of American office workers usually eat their lunch in the same spot they work all day.' Captions include: 'Cold spaghetti bolognese. Eaten with a spoon. #sigh' and 'I almost skipped lunch rather than eat this.'

Finally, on Instagram we have the account Cooking for Bae (@cookingforbae), which reposts the most horrifyingly unappetising meals someone has cooked for their partner. This account has become so popular that some people have sent in intentionally ugly food. This isn't allowed, as the food has to be real. The vast majority of the contributions have been sent in by people without their partner's knowledge, although one or two have spotted their creations and complained. Like the other accounts, the food is seriously unattractive and definitely grounds for dumping someone.

Perfectly imperfect

While there is certainly an increased backlash against the culture of perfectionism online, and some of it has been very needed, it feels as though this has also created a new pressure: to be perfectly imperfect. You must embrace your flaws, but only if they are near-universally accepted. Show us your stretch marks and scars, as long as they are on a thin body and not self-inflicted. Talk about your anxiety, sure, but please keep your 'less palatable' borderline personality disorder to yourself. Post your ironic 'Instagram vs reality' posts, but still present them beautifully and edit them to look appealing. Oh, and make sure you're thin, otherwise it's just 'gross'.

We want our online experts to share that they're 'still on this journey' while giving us perfect advice that will always help, never harm, and is exactly what we want to hear. And, above all, it must be presented to us in a perfectly edited but 'natural' way. It has to be #authentic.

We have huge expectations on us to achieve perfection by ourselves, others, society or a combination of the three. The better you do, the better you're expected to be. Once you meet a certain standard you're expected either to match or exceed it. Yet, even if we meet these high standards, that isn't guarantee enough. We ask ourselves 'how can I be a success when I'm having to try so much harder than others to achieve the same outcomes?' It's not enough to reach that impossibly high standard, it also has to appear effortless. Unsurprisingly, this can have a negative impact on our health, which we'll explore in the next chapter.

6

WHAT IMPACT IS SOCIAL MEDIA HAVING ON MY HEALTH?

You'll notice that so far several of the chapter subjects inter-link. The concept of the 'perfect' diet can lead to shaming of others for their food choices when they are perceived as 'not good enough'. The influence that online personas can have over our food choices can lead us down the path of food extremism. All of these can drive food anxieties and uncertainty around food. They can also lead to our health and wellbeing becoming negatively affected.

The most obvious and well-known links are between social media use and mental health issues such as depression, anxiety and eating disorders. While the last of these is clearly related to food, all mental health conditions can have a connection to food and eating in some way. Even when not specifically food-related, I still feel it is important to talk about social media in the context of our overall health, with an additional focus on food.

Social media is the bubble with which we surround ourselves. We can choose who we follow and, in theory, how much time we spend on it, but when we make those choices we often stick with our echo chamber and don't seek out alternate opinions. We often need a variety of views to be able to make an informed, educated decision. When you consider this in relation to health or self-worth, social media therefore has the potential to be incredibly dangerous.

What often mediates this relationship between social media and poor mental health is social comparison. As a reminder: comparison can be upward or downward. Upward social comparison occurs when we compare ourselves to those who are similar but slightly better than us at something, whereas downward social comparison occurs when we compare ourselves to those who are slightly worse. Although upward social comparison can be beneficial and drive us to do better, more often than not it causes us to feel inadequate.

Overall, while real-world social interactions are linked to better overall wellbeing, using social media like Facebook can have the opposite effect. This is particularly so when it comes to mental health, as most measures of Facebook use predict a decrease in mental health after a year, as well as poorer physical health and life satisfaction. It doesn't matter if you're liking other people's content, or crafting your own tweet or status update, quantity as well as quality of time spent online can be detrimental.

Depression and anxiety

We know that spending large amounts of time on social media is associated with depression and anxiety. What is also relevant is the number of social media platforms you use. Compared to those who use 0-2 social media platforms, for people who use 7-11 platforms the odds of having greater symptoms of both depression and anxiety are substantially higher. This may partly be explained by the likelihood that individuals who spend a lot of time online may be substituting social media for face-to-face social interactions. Frequent exposure to highly curated, unrealistic portrayals on social media that give the impression that others are living happier, more connected lives, may make people feel more socially isolated and lonely.

Self-esteem

Self-esteem refers to a person's positive or negative evaluation of the self. In other words, it's the extent to which someone views themselves as worthwhile and competent. Self-esteem can be both a stable trait that develops over time, as well as a fluid state that responds to daily events. Regular and repeated exposure to upward social comparisons on social media can have a negative impact on people's self-esteem.

Research shows that people who had the most chronic exposure to Facebook (meaning they used it most frequently) tended to have lower self-esteem. We all spend far more time engaging in upward, rather than downward, social comparison on Facebook, and these upward social comparisons are the underlying reason why social media can lower people's self-esteem – regular comparison really does make you feel shit.

Essentially, the more time you spend on Facebook, the more likely you are to make upward social comparisons, and the lower your self-esteem may sink. This occurs both immediately in response to individual posts, and long term with repeated exposure.

The number of likes an individual receives on their Facebook profile pictures is positively associated with self-esteem, but only temporarily. A lack of engagement, on the other hand, can create a drop in our self-esteem. Research suggests that if your self-esteem was low to begin with, a lack of engagement on social media is more likely to negatively affect you. So the people who feel the strongest need for validation are also those who are least able to cope with the negative effects of low engagement online. Those people with low self-esteem are far more vulnerable to being jolted about by the effects of likes and comments, with a higher chance of experiencing both highs and lows.

Of course, this outcome isn't unique to Facebook, but it seems to be more pronounced on Facebook and Instagram compared to other platforms.

Body image and disordered eating

Body image is the compilation of a person's thoughts, perceptions and feelings about their body. Poor body image, or body dissatisfaction, is so common now that up to 80% of women and 50% of men are unhappy with their bodies. Rates of body dissatisfaction are reported to be even higher in the transgender community due to gender dysphoria. This discontentment can develop from as early as six years old, and can last a lifetime, while leading to those familiar issues of depression, anxiety and eating disorders.

We've long known the impact media images can have on how we view our bodies. We're presented on a daily basis with idealised images of how we *should* look, images that are impossible for most of us to reach. When we inevitably fail to achieve this ideal, we engage in comparison where we fall short, resulting in a sense of dissatisfaction in the body we occupy. We feel disappointment, frustration, anxiety and shame.

Now we also have social media, which allows us to make comparisons not just with celebrities and models who are so unlike us, but also to Instagram models, influencers and friends. These comparisons are arguably much more powerful because we feel these people are truly our peers: they don't have a huge team of people they pay to make them look this way (nutritionists, personal trainers, chefs, etc.), they're normal people just like us! Except, often they're not.

Research shows that spending more time on social media is associated with more body-checking, higher endorsement for unrealistic body ideals, higher levels of body comparison, greater weight dissatisfaction and more disordered eating. Social media use is a predictor of body image and eating concerns up to eighteen months down the line. In other words, your social media use now can predict how dissatisfied you'll be with your body and eating over a year into the future.

One of the latest body trends on social media has been more along the lines of 'strong not skinny', which has prematurely been hailed as a good thing for women. I beg to differ. What we really mean is 'strong *and* skinny', because strong and fat is still seen as being far from the ideal body. Rather than change the ideal body standards, it's simply added another aspect to aim for. And let's face it, a lot of these popular #fitspo bloggers would look almost exactly the same even if they rarely went to the gym. I've seen the before and after pictures they post, and sometimes even when I squint I struggle to see any real difference. The truth is these women are often naturally long and lean and now just look long and lean but with better lighting and tensed muscles. Social media definitely seems to have upped the level of muscle tone that's now considered to be necessary for the ideal body.

Disliking yourself is non-discriminatory

There is a common misconception that body dissatisfaction is purely a female issue, and while the conversation and research are definitely focused there, it is something that affects all genders.

Men may not have the same pressure to be thin but the lean body ideal still exists, and has become increasingly muscular over time (think *Men's Health* cover, or Marvel superheroes). In fact, the ideal male body marketed to men is more muscular than the ideal male body marketed to women. In general, men over-estimate the degree of muscularity that is attractive to women, and women overestimate the degree of thinness that is attractive to men. As a result, the images of men in men's magazines are more muscular than those in women's magazines.

The impact of ideal media images may be seen in the increasing prevalence of eating disorder symptoms, body dysmorphia, excessive exercise, and steroid use among men. A lot of the inspirational images of the 'ideal' man are very much in the realm of #fitspo – very lean and very muscular.

Transgender and gender non-conforming (TGNC) individuals are at a higher risk of mental health issues, such as depression, suicidal thoughts, self-injury, body dissatisfaction and eating disorders. The reasons for this are generally attributed to the huge discrimination and abuse to which these identities are exposed by the public at large, in the media, and often even by family members.

This is a group of people that is incredibly underrepresented in research, and while I couldn't find any papers specifically on social media and TGNC folk, based on my own clinical practice and conversations with TGNC individuals I'd like to make some predictions. I can see the role of social media going two ways: either the community aspect of social media and seeing amazing TGNC bodies being unashamedly themselves could be a protective factor; or I could see the popularity of trans people who very much conform to gender stereotypes being an additional risk factor for body dissatisfaction. The main reason for the former scenario comes from the fact that social connectedness and support are known to be protective against depression and anxiety in TGNC folks and can help foster resilience to discrimination. The latter comes from knowledge of what society deems to be beautiful and acceptable for human bodies to look like.

Feminist scholars have long argued that women are taught to view their bodies as an outsider would, constantly considering how attractive their bodies are to a (male) observer. Any woman who's ever walked down a busy street and been catcalled knows exactly what this 'male gaze' feels like. This gaze has an effect on women's body image because they are encouraged to try and transform their bodies into something that fits what men find desirable, rather than what they actually want. This is known as 'objectification theory' – where women in particular are taught to see their bodies as objects for consumption. Objectification theory is supported by an abundance of research documenting the link between objectification experiences and self-objectification (where you start to view your body as an object because it's so reinforced through experience with others), as well as the link between self-objectification and disordered eating. Obviously, this occurs mainly in heterosexual women as they are trying to seek a male partner.

This theory also helps to explain why gay and bisexual men are more prone to disordered eating, as they too, in some shape or form, are catering to a male gaze. Lesbian women, on the other hand, tend to be more protected from this, and as such have lower rates of body dissatisfaction and disordered eating. Interestingly, bisexual women were found to be more dissatisfied with their body image and to have a higher incidence of unhealthy weight control practices than lesbians and heterosexual women.* As with TGNC people, being part of a supportive and inclusive LGBTQ+ community, either in person or online through social media, can be a protective factor against body dissatisfaction and disordered eating.

Who do we blame?

Ultimately, social media is neither a cause nor an effect of disordered eating, but it can play a pivotal role in our complex

---

* There are a number of potential reasons for this; unfortunately I don't have space to delve into these thoroughly. If you're keen to read more, check out the paper by Chmielewski and Yost in the bibliography.

relationship with food. Like food, social media is at once a private and public experience: we can consume it alone, but it always connects us to others. In the most extreme cases, social media can provide a haven for 'pro-ana' content, which actively promotes eating disorders such as anorexia nervosa as a legitimate lifestyle that should be encouraged. Users share tips and tricks, with the express wish of avoiding recovery. It's truly heart-breaking. Thankfully, there has been a significant crackdown by social media platforms on this kind of content, although it still manages to seep in. And, of course, with orthorexia, it's often encouraged by unsuspecting followers.

The emergence of orthorexia in particular has occurred alongside an exploding wellness industry, featuring a mix of actual experts with sensible advice and a plethora of charlatans preying on people's insecurities. Fitspos, alternative therapies, cleanses, health magazines... all using social media to showcase 'perfect bodies' and 'perfect eating' and, of course, all under the guise of inspiration and female empowerment.

The 'clean eating' revolution has been intensely amplified by the digital revolution – and naturally Instagram is/was the platform of choice for 'clean eating'. The entire notion of clean eating – of overly moralised food choices, of purity attached to eating – inevitably led to a rise in anxiety around eating and to a rise in orthorexia. Looking back, I can't muster up any surprise that the consequences for people's health were negative.

Rebecca, currently in recovery from an eating disorder, shared with me how social media played (and still continues to play) a role in her health issues: "In my experience, social media has fuelled my eating disorder by creating an aspirational, unachievable ideal diet and body shape. I see beautiful, desirable meals

that are generally vegan, which I compare to my own meals. It is
this comparison that makes your food choices seem inadequate,
so you aspire to make food that is 'Instagram-worthy'. Repeated
messages about the food you *should* be eating (particularly no
refined sugar or animal products) means that these 'rules' are
ingrained and led me to continue feeling guilty if I didn't abide
by them. I do have quite a bit of knowledge around nutrition
(not just due to my eating disorder, although of course that did
assist in my thirst for knowledge) so am aware that lots of the
messages online are false, yet I am still drawn into them and I
think this shows the power of social media and how influential
those who post on social media are. In terms of body image,
social media means that you see unrealistic body images through
Photoshopping but also from those who may be underweight
posting images of their bodies. Without proper censoring on
social media, you just end up seeing bodies that are not healthy
to aspire to, or are not even achievable at all but just the work
of a computer. I know that these images have had a massive
impact on the development of my eating disorder and also in
the hindrance of my recovery because they made me see my
own body as wrong, which no one should ever feel. Somehow,
social media raises the unqualified into positions of influence
which leads to distorted messages being sent out to the public.
The ability to make images very aesthetically pleasing just means
that you are more drawn to them, independent of the validity
of their claims."

I've observed an interesting pattern when it comes to social
media and disordered eating. Many people have reached out to
me and shared that platforms like Instagram enabled their disordered habits through the people they were following, but once

they unfollowed the negative influences and replaced them with professionals and recovery accounts, Instagram helped them persevere through recovery to a happier place with food. Michelle Elman, for example, gives credit to social media for opening her eyes about her relationship with food: "Social media was actually where I first realised that I had disordered eating habits and discovered what diet culture was. There was no conversation taking place outside of social media where I could have found out this information because it was unthinkable that I could have restrictive behaviours and be fat."

So far in this book we have discussed how social media shapes the way we eat through various mechanisms: social comparison, impression management, extremism, perfectionism and shame. These mechanisms can help explain the link between social media use and poor health outcomes, especially poor mental health. The rest of this chapter aims to link the ideas I've discussed so far to the mental health impacts social media can have, and explain the extent of the effect these concepts have on how we feel.

Who decides what you eat?

There are many examples of social media wellness influencers who have transformed followers into a lucrative career, among them Belle Gibson, Freelee the Banana Girl, David 'Avocado' Wolfe... weirdly, all people I hate. While these people have some mainstream media success, it's the large free platforms offered by social media that provide the key to their success. It's no coincidence that the popularity of these wellness influencers is matched by a rise in eating disorders.

In our current social media landscape of idealised bodies, perfectly Instagrammed food, and a dominant narrative of taking control and ownership over your health, there is no shortage of models that someone may follow down an orthorexic path. Where the successful blogger or Instagram influencer (Jordan Younger, for instance) engages in the performance of health online, their thousands of followers then engage in a copycat performance, taking their own health to a potentially extreme, obsessive place.

These influencers primarily engage in transactional relationships with others, they have followers rather than friends, and even people they call 'friends' are often strategic partnerships to boost each other's online profiles.

As the term suggests, influencers have huge power and responsibility, even if they have no qualifications, and people will listen to them and copy what they do. Most of the popular food and health influencers are notably thin and claim that their way of eating is either the 'perfect' way to eat, is guaranteed to make someone healthier, or will cure everything under the sun.

Sounds pretty extreme.

How extreme are your choices?

It's clear that extreme patterns of eating are inherently quite restrictive and therefore may lead to nutritional deficiencies. For example, any form of veganism, whether it's raw vegan, fruitarian or just standard vegan, requires the supplementation of vitamin B12. A very low-carbohydrate diet such as keto could easily be low in fibre and high in saturated fat, a pattern we know increases risk of heart disease. And, of course, the complete elimination of all plant foods through a carnivore diet carries so many risks, not least vitamin C deficiency, also known as scurvy.

The pattern of harm seems to be this: the vegan side is far more likely to result in psychological harm. Vegans are over-represented in eating disorder treatment centres – only around 1% of the UK population is vegan but they represent a far greater percentage of patients with eating disorders. On the low-carb side, on the other hand, the harm is far more likely to be physiological, through a dismissal of the importance of fibre and promoting the idea that saturated fat is harmless, which we definitely know is not true.

Recently, we've also seen the rise of another concerning movement – the 'Food is Medicine' crew. This is a group of (primarily) doctors who are keen to learn more about nutrition and have more nutrition training in medical schools – very admirable goals – but with a frightening misunderstanding of the role of food in health. Food is not medicine. The two are not equivalent. Nutrition is primarily preventative rather than a cure. A high-fibre diet, for example, can be protective against some cancers, but is beyond useless if you already have cancer. Even the word 'prevent' here can be misleading, because you can have the 'perfect' diet and still develop cancer, heart disease or dementia. Food is never guaranteed to prevent a chronic condition, because these conditions are incredibly complex, but it can contribute to decreasing your risk over the course of your life. What this 'Food is Medicine' narrative does, though, is place the blame back on the individual with the disease, when that is neither accurate nor helpful. It's food shaming.

A common interpretation of this is the idea that if you say food is no guarantee that you won't become unwell, that you could have the best diet in the world and still get cancer, then it encourages people to not give a shit about what they eat. I completely reject this false dichotomy. It's not one or the other, there are plenty of nuanced alternatives. Food isn't guaranteed to prevent heart disease; however, you can still reduce your risk by eating plenty of fibre. No shame and judgement, no unrealistic statements. Of course food still matters, but it's important to put it into context and not see it as some miracle.

Food operates within specific roles and biomedical parameters, whereas the very nature of pharmaceutical drugs and other medicines is that the dosage is on an entirely different level. It operates outside the biological range of food – that's what makes it medicine. It's been purified and concentrated to provide a therapeutic dose.

The big issue with the 'Food is Medicine' rhetoric is that it is too easily interpreted as 'use food *instead* of medicine'. When people are choosing food over proven effective conventional medical treatment, that is a huge cause for concern.

I really do believe that the vast majority of doctors in this space are coming from a good place, that they don't mean harm. But that's just not good enough. Often they're saying that food can be useful in addition to medication to help your condition, but that message appears alongside quacks who say to use food instead of medicine to treat your condition, and by using the same phrase – 'Food is Medicine' – the former inadvertently encourage people to listen to the latter.

You'll commonly hear the 'Food is Medicine' doctors sharing recipes using foods they claim have 'medicinal properties'. For example: vitamin A is important for eyesight. Carrots contain beta-carotene (a plant form of vitamin A), therefore this carrot curry will make your eyesight better. That's not how it works. According to them, 'it's just food, what's the harm?'

Here's the harm: we are now seeing an increase in people refusing medical treatment options to opt for 'Food is Medicine' instead. People are refusing chemotherapy to take turmeric supplements or high-dose intravenous vitamin drips. While the quacks may be the ones encouraging turmeric, what the 'Food is Medicine' legitimate doctors don't understand is that their rhetoric is encouraging this behaviour whether they like it or not. When your catchphrase is being used to push harmful information, you have to let that shit go to distance yourself and prevent further harm.

The hardcore quacks parroting this phrase use social media to encourage people to 'heal naturally' rather than using medication or other traditional medicine. For example, P (see pages 128–31) has received many Instagram DMs from people saying they should heal their acne naturally. Karl* was diagnosed with depression as a teenager, and says, "I become interested in 'healing' myself 'naturally' when I was put on anti-depressants after I had a mental breakdown. I had heard some people say that this could be done with food rather than medication, so I thought I'd look into it and that's when I started to compare my diet to others. It made me hyper-aware of my food and often insecure when I didn't feel like I lived up to what I thought would have been expected of me if I knew/were friends with the people I followed." This had a significant impact on Karl's wellbeing.

* Name changed.

"It affected me mentally as I tried not taking my meds and I became very depressed again, very quickly. It also formed an obsession with food that made it really hard to enjoy food when I didn't have control, and I come from a family where food is very social, so it was difficult to be social when I was so convinced I had to eat/not eat certain foods."

In its extreme form, the 'Food is Medicine' rhetoric drives people towards quack therapies such as Gerson therapy. This is a treatment protocol that claims to allow the body to heal itself using 'an organic, plant-based diet, raw juices, coffee enemas and natural supplements'. Let me state right from the start that it absolutely doesn't.

In 2008 Jess Ainscough was told she had an incredibly rare form of cancer known as epithelioid sarcoma. She was just 22 years old. Her doctor recommended that her arm, and possibly also her shoulder, be amputated. Instead, she decided to follow Gerson therapy. She wrote: "The way I saw it I had two choices. I could let them chase the disease around my body until there was nothing left of me to cut, zap or poison; or I could take responsibility for my illness and bring my body to optimum health so that it can heal itself. For me it was an easy decision." She wrote about this regularly on her blog, and gained the name the Wellness Warrior. Jess spent a few weeks in the Gerson clinic in Tijuana – a city in Mexico, just south of the border with California – before spending the next two years continuing this protocol at home.

About a year after Jess started Gerson therapy, she wrote that her mother Sharyn was diagnosed with breast cancer and began following the same treatment. Sadly, Sharyn died around two and a half years later, which is close to the known median survival of untreated breast cancer. It's unclear who influenced who to start following alternative therapies, but what is clear is that Sharyn died unnecessarily. Sadly, in February 2015, Jess Ainscough also died. While her death shows she was undoubtedly a victim of extreme pseudoscience, it's uncertain how many others suffered because of her promotion of Gerson. Whenever someone says 'it's just celery juice, what's the harm?', this story always comes to mind.

Pro-ana forums, while once focused purely on calories, are now just as fixated on extreme diets as wellness gurus on social media. The same influencers who are praised for their healthfulness on Instagram are also being hailed as 'thinspiration' on pro-ana forums. Raw til Four, 30 Bananas a Day, and the ketogenic diet all have their own discussion threads. These extreme diets are praised for the way they can be used to mask disordered eating behaviour, turning obsession into a more socially acceptable form.

While we cannot blame social media as the sole cause of food obsessions and eating disorders, we cannot deny the role it can play in triggering disordered thoughts or delaying recovery. Rebecca, who we heard from earlier, says that although her eating disorder was in full force before she joined Instagram, the algorithm has made her recovery more challenging: "The thing with social media is that, even if you unfollow certain 'triggering' accounts, your search history will still mean that these kinds of accounts are recommended to you to follow. I often still find myself drawn into the matrix of Instagram accounts and, once again, idealising different eating habits that I know to be 'unhealthy' and unattainable."

In 2016, eating disorder psychiatrist Dr Mark Berelowitz said a shocking 80–90% of patients attending his North London clinic were avid followers of bloggers and social media influencers who advised avoiding entire food groups, including sugar. I can say the same thing about my own clinic, which is frightening.

What is your image curation doing to you?

One of the big appeals of social media platforms is that they allow us to curate a particular public image and have considerable control over the image we choose to present to the world. Yet this new avenue of impression management has not eased our anxiety. Instead, this exposure to others' perfect self-representations on social media can lead us to fixate on our own body dissatisfaction and lack of social life. Our minds are struggling to cope with this 24/7 access to visuals that emphasise unrealistic and (for the vast majority of us) unattainable body ideals. The most recent cohort data from the United States and the United Kingdom show that incidences of body dysmorphia and eating disorders have risen by approximately 30% among adolescents since the rise of social media. In the same countries, increasing numbers of young people are responding to this pressure to look perfect by turning to plastic surgery and its promise of bodily perfection.

It seems that this control and curation, for the most part, is adding an additional source of stress, anxiety and comparison to our lives. Before social media we would most likely just go home, go about our business without anyone watching (even virtually), then come back into school or work the next day having had a break. Now, we take the external gaze home with us.

This also helps to explain why using a large number of social media platforms, rather than just one or two, is more linked to depression and anxiety. Using multiple platforms can lead to identity diffusion – where someone hasn't committed to an identity and isn't working to form one – possibly because they're a slightly different version of themselves on each platform. If you're a different person in each setting, and you're switching between them, your sense of self can be fragmented, and you don't know which version is the true you. This fragmentation isn't 'fake' in the strictest sense of the word, just carefully selected parts of an incomplete picture.

Chronic dieters and individuals struggling with eating disorders are more likely to be influenced by food-related impression management, especially in the context of judgements about body size and weight. Research suggests that these people believe that a high-fat diet has a much greater impact on someone's weight than those with healthier relationships with food. The food doesn't actually have a greater impact on their weight, but they truly believe it would. This is based on the common phrase 'fat makes you fat', which is in itself a consumption stereotype. Note that restrictive eaters do not just apply this idea to themselves but also to others. In fact, there's evidence that they're more likely to make judgements about other people's body weight based on their food intake.

These stereotypes also contribute to how restrictive and restrained eaters feel about their bodies. Individuals with bulimia tend to perceive themselves to be heavier after eating a chocolate bar, and those with disordered eating symptoms perceive themselves to have gained weight after simply imagining that they have consumed a 'bad' or forbidden food. In this way, they may be using restrictive eating as a way to feel better about their own body image, which can lead to maintenance of restrictive behaviours and prevent recovery. These ideas can affect the person's behaviour, as well as potentially what they post online.

For most of us, we know we can't deceive ourselves, but at least we can have an impact on how others perceive us. However, this comes with the downside of a double standard. Even though we know the images we post of ourselves online aren't a complete representation of us as a person, we still struggle to remind ourselves to apply this logic to others, which makes that comparison so much easier to do.

It's also important to highlight that curating an online social media persona different from your everyday life *can* be a good thing. For example, LGBTQ+ people who are afraid to come out to friends or family can find an LGBTQ+ community online who can reassure them that they are not broken or wrong in some way, and can help with the process of navigating their identity, either for themselves or in relation to family and friends. Or if you really love cooking or baking but none of your friends is interested, then sharing your images online and receiving praise from strangers can be an additional motivator to keep going and pursue your passion. Of course, we should be aiming for internal validation (from within ourselves), but it's easier said than done, and external validation from others does make life simpler.

Having this online version of yourself can be beneficial to begin with, absolutely, but care needs to be taken that this disconnect between online and offline doesn't become an additional source of stress, either due to the fear of being 'found out' or because of the pressure to be perfect.

How perfect is too perfect?

Speaking of perfectionism, so far we've mainly spoken about perfectionism in the context of the quest for the 'perfect' diet progressing into orthorexia. Aside from orthorexia, perfectionism also has additional consequences related to mental health. According to the American Psychological Association, perfectionism among young people has significantly increased since the 1980s. This rise in perfectionism is said to be contributing to an increase in stress, depression and anxiety.

Perfectionistic self-promoters might promote a version of themselves that is, well, perfect, and focused on their positive attributes when interacting with others. This isn't narcissism but is a perfectionist's way of attempting to gain admiration and respect from others. They present themselves as a good person, dedicated, kind and successful in every aspect of life. Such perfectionistic self-presentation is linked to lower self-esteem and higher risk of depression. On social media in particular, it's linked to higher stress and risk of anxiety.

Perfectionism has long been linked to eating disorders. It feels like one of the more obvious links, as seeking total perfection includes seeking the 'perfect' body, which has to be managed through food. Eating-disorder pioneer Hilde Bruch characterised young patients with anorexia nervosa as fulfilling "every parent's and teacher's idea of perfection". By this she meant that young people with anorexia can often be people-pleasers trying to keep everyone around them happy. They may be striving to get exceptional grades and may always be compliant, never complaining or confronting their parents or teachers. In other words, what could be perceived as the 'ideal' child or student.

It has been suggested that the common central features of both anorexia and bulimia, particularly this striving for a 'perfect' body shape, are inherently perfectionistic.

Children and adolescents who score highly on scales of perfectionism are far more likely to develop disordered eating or an eating disorder, particularly anorexia nervosa. Around 70% of people with anorexia score highly on socially prescribed perfectionism, and around 90% score highly on self-oriented perfectionism. Perfectionism acts together with low self-esteem and poor body image to raise someone's risk of an eating disorder, and also seems to make recovery more challenging. Those who have recovered from an eating disorder still often have higher levels of perfectionism than the general population, even for up to twelve years after the initial diagnosis. This is likely a symptom of the over-reliance on physical indicators of recovery and a lack of focus on psychological indicators, which need to be seen as equally important.

Individuals with an eating disorder are often not simply perfectionists when it comes to food, weight and shape, but also in other domains of life. For example, individuals may be over-achievers at school, play large amounts of sports, or worry excessively about being the perfect friend. It is rare for someone to have perfectionistic tendencies when it comes to food and nothing else.

Of the many components of perfectionism, the obsessional aspect of perfectionism that drives excessive concern over mistakes, as well as doubts about actions (including the ability to complete tasks), has the strongest association with eating disorders. Doubts and anxieties about completing tasks correctly are associated with both eating disorders and anxiety, which helps explain why a high percentage of individuals with eating disorders report co-morbid anxiety disorders, which tend to persist even after someone has recovered (or is deemed to have recovered) from an eating disorder.

One possible mechanism that explains the link between perfectionism and eating disorders is that maladaptive perfectionism involves doubts about behaviour, excessive concerns over making mistakes, and a heightened sensitivity to the expectations of others. These can be hard to objectively quantify as they aren't easily tangible, leading perfectionists to find more concrete sources of validation such as social comparison (which is rife on social media) or a focus on the number on the bathroom scales. Losing weight often leads to praise and validation from others, which can feel a more reliable aim. When we factor in the huge amount of comparison available to us online, and the fact that socially prescribed perfectionism is linked to body image concerns, this seems to fit.

Most concerningly, the desire to be perfect has even been tied to suicidal thoughts. In a meta-analysis published in 2017, researchers found evidence to link perfectionism to suicidal thoughts and behaviours. Both self-oriented and socially prescribed perfectionism are linked to suicidal tendencies – self-oriented perfectionism predicts suicide ideation (suicidal thoughts), while socially prescribed perfectionism predicts suicide ideation and actual attempts.

So, why is perfectionism associated with thinking about, attempting and even completing suicide? Perfectionists are often their own worst critics, they are never good enough, and never satisfied with their achievements. Perfectionists can therefore become locked in an endless loop of self-defeating striving for impossible goals in which each new task is another opportunity for harsh self-criticism, disappointment and failure. In addition, black-and-white thinking is a key pattern in perfectionists, and leads perfectionists to interpret failures as catastrophes that, in extreme circumstances, are seen as warranting death. 'If I fail, then I don't deserve to live' may feel like a dramatic statement to many of us, but these thought patterns are incredibly powerful, especially when the shame of failure causes people to hide their thoughts from others.

Perfectionism is increasingly being seen as a risk factor for suicide that has a double-edged sword. Perfectionists tend to have extremely high expectations of themselves and engage in severe self-criticism and black-and-white thinking when they fail to meet these standards. They also have a tendency to show a 'perfect face' to the world to maintain the illusion of perfection, so they won't have failed in the eyes of others. These two factors together increase someone's risk of suicide ideation while decreasing the likelihood they will seek help when they should. Social media can be a significant contributor to the pressure to achieve and maintain impossibly perfect standards, and to maintain the impression of being perfect in the eyes of others.

When people experience their social world as pressure-filled, judgemental and hypercritical, they are far more likely to consider or engage in potential means of escape, such as alcohol misuse, disordered eating and suicide. That social world can be online, offline or both.

Overall, while there's nothing wrong with wanting to show yourself from your best angle, it's important that we still like ourselves when we're not looking our best, which, let's be honest, is probably a decent amount of the time. It's also important that we acknowledge the absence of the 'perfect diet' – it simply does not exist. Food is complex, individual and variable. It's even more important that we recognise the potential for social media to exacerbate and enable perfectionistic thinking, regarding food or other aspects of our lives.

How bad is shaming?

Food shaming is inextricably linked with body shaming, and while shaming in any context can be harmful, when it comes to health it seems shame may even be a *direct cause* of ill health. As a quick reminder, shame is not the same as guilt: guilt is related to action and having done something wrong, whereas shame is related to feeling judged by others to be flawed, inadequate or wrong in some way. Guilt is the feeling of doing wrong, whereas shame is the feeling of *being* wrong. I firmly believe that feeling guilty for eating, something we need to do in order to survive, is something we need to remove from our consciousness, but shame is on a whole other level. Because shame is linked to our core identity, it is among the most powerful and significant emotional experiences. On top of that, it is seen as shameful to feel shame, which leads us to avoid and deny our own emotional experiences.

While experiences of shaming regarding food and health can produce feelings of inadequacy, there is so much more to it than this. Shame impacts on health through a variety of interrelated pathways: via acute and chronic shame avoidance behaviour, and biological mechanisms.

Acute shame is a single, isolated experience of shame. It is uncomfortable, and from a health perspective usually results from exposing a perceived flaw, which could be overeating, becoming ill, skipping a few fitness classes, or developing some marker that could be seen as unattractive, for example acne or a rash. We may deliberately hide these from others, including on social media, to avoid the experience of shame or being shamed. In a healthcare setting this can mean a delay in seeking treatment, and online it can produce a building anxiety about being 'found out'.

Chronic shame is a persistent pattern that can be present throughout someone's entire life. This is more likely to occur when there is a fear of being shamed for some part of yourself that is constant or near-constant over time, for example your sexuality, gender identity, childhood traumas and other adverse experiences, or weight. There is a growing body of work that shows people who experience chronic shame are more likely to engage in risk behaviours such as alcoholism, addiction and eating disorders, all of which act to 'numb' an individual against the pain of shame. In a social media setting, it can lead people to feel the need to keep these aspects of themselves secret, not simply because they want to (which is perfectly within their rights), but because they feel they have to. As we have seen in the section on impression management (see pages 51–5), that discrepancy between the true self and the online self can be incredibly stressful.

Experiences of shame cause prolonged stress in the body, which has a clear effect on many physiological systems, such as the immune and cardiovascular systems. Threats to self-esteem or social status, also known as social-evaluative threats, can lead to increased anxiety and a stronger stress response. The biological response to stress includes the release of the hormone cortisol and inflammatory markers into the bloodstream, similar to the 'fight or flight' response. To be clear: occasional doses of shame may feel awful in that moment but are a part of being human and are not harmful in the long term. However, when this is a regular or chronic occurrence it can result in wear and tear of the immune system, as well as an increased risk of heart disease.

Shame can also drive psychological issues, such as depression. When we regularly experience shame, we reinforce the narrative that we *are* wrong, and that these flaws are deeply within us, rather than related to something we have done. When this is perpetuated, it can lead to a deep sense of being inadequate, not good enough, not worthy. Depression, and its accompanying feeling of lethargy and hopelessness, can further drive shame and thoughts of 'I can't do anything right', 'I'm such a failure' and 'I'm an idiot', leading to a shame spiral that's difficult to escape from.

Jon Ronson, the absolute genius, wrote a book titled *So You've Been Publicly Shamed*. If you haven't read it I highly recommend it, as it's really an incredible read. In this book, Jon writes about instances where individuals have been publicly shamed on social media to the point where they have lost their jobs, lost friends, and/or been dumped. In short: their lives have sometimes been completely ruined by the shame pile-on in response to a single tweet.

It's not all in your head

I'm loath to separate this into the categories of 'mental' versus 'physical' health, as the two are inextricably interlinked, and one will influence the other. However, where the research has focused purely on the physical health effects of social media, it has tended towards sedentary behaviour and overeating.

Research has shown that using social media may detract from face-to-face relationships, reduce investment in meaningful activities, and increase sedentary behaviour by encouraging more screen time. The biggest issue here with excessive social media use is that it displaces other activities. If people are using their phones so much that it's replacing time outdoors or time moving their bodies, then that can have a negative impact. We know that sedentary behaviour is associated with greater risk of several major chronic disease outcomes, including heart disease, type-2 diabetes and cancer, particularly above 6–8 hours per day of total sitting.

There is also some concern about distracted eating when watching screens and scrolling through social media, which can take the focus away from the body's intuitive signs of fullness, thereby making it easier to accidently overeat past comfortable fullness.

In one 2017 survey conducted in the UK, 55% of respondents said they look at their phone within 15 minutes of waking and 28% check their phone within 5 minutes of attempting to sleep, every night, thereby exposing themselves to bright blue light which can impact their quality of sleep. Every night. In addition, 40% said they weren't going to bed at the intended time because of their phone, while 13% wake up at night to check their phone.

High Internet usage is associated with shorter sleep duration, later sleep time, difficulty getting to sleep, and being tired during the day, especially among adolescents. Another survey of young people found that 37% reported losing sleep due to spending time on social media in bed. Social media has a uniquely detrimental effect on sleep because alerts at night can disturb sleep (and many people sleep with the phone next to or under their pillow), and incoming alerts can create pressure to be available at all hours to respond to people, or potentially miss out. Overall, high social media use, high night-time social media use, and emotional investment in social media are all linked to poor sleep, greater risk of depression and anxiety, and lower self-esteem.

Disrupting sleep and reducing sleep time is obviously an issue, as sleep is one of the basic needs for human survival. If you don't sleep, you die, and, generally speaking, the less you sleep, the sooner you die. The effects of insufficient sleep are pretty severe: dampened immune system, disruption of blood sugar levels, reduced concentration, impaired memory, and increased risk of cancer, heart disease, stroke, dementia, depression and anxiety. That's a lot of unwelcome consequences. Lack of sleep also disrupts your hunger hormones, which makes you feel hungrier the next day, less satisfied with the same amount of food, and with stronger cravings for comfort food. Not an issue if it's every once in a while, but it can potentially become a problem over long periods of time.

There are a lot of media scare stories about how we're all becoming lonelier even though, virtually, we're more connected than ever before. There is an element of truth to this, but it partly depends on how you're using social media. If you're passively scrolling without engaging, or just posting and disappearing, or simply hitting the like button then, yes, this will likely have a harmful effect in terms of comparison and loneliness. However, if you're actively engaging with people in a meaningful way and having genuine conversations, that's a whole other scenario.

The full story when it comes to online social media relationships is complex. I'm an example of someone who met many of her closest friends online. I met one of my best friends on a forum when we were both 15, and we would chat every night on MSN Messenger,* and now, as an adult, some of the people who make my life undoubtedly better became close friends of mine through Instagram and Twitter. The key, though, is that while we may have met online, we spend plenty of time together face to face, and those in-person interactions are always far more rewarding and enjoyable. Social media can give an illusion of meaningful social interaction, but it can also be truly meaningful, especially if it's in addition to an in-person relationship, leads to an in-person relationship, or meeting face to face isn't feasible.

Social media is intended to be social, and when we use social media to have supportive interactions, we see that people are generally happier after. The number of friends you have on Facebook or followers on Twitter or Instagram doesn't really matter, it's how you communicate with these people that is important. Being sociable and getting support from others is one of the key factors to human longevity and life satisfaction. Although social media does help people to expand their network, this network is only valid if it provides the social support and sense of community that we need.

In the context of food, this community can be particularly important. Perhaps you're living with type-1 diabetes and no one else in your town is. Or you're the only ethical vegan in your family. Or you have coeliac disease and have no idea how to cook delicious gluten-free meals for yourself. In those scenarios,

---

* Just typing that makes me feel old.

social media can be a hugely positive influence. And even if those don't apply to you, social media can still be a supportive online community that makes you happy.

For example, blogger and content creator Becky Excell says, "Social media has definitely helped the most with discovering products that are suitable for my dietary issues. Brands use social media to push out new gluten-free products regularly, and as a community we all share product finds regularly to help each other. And within the gluten-free and IBS community online there is a lot of sharing of personal experiences. I do find this helps in terms of making me (and others) feel less alone when having a really bad day."

Social media has far-reaching impacts on our mental, physical and social health. Many of its effects are clearly negative, and it can contribute to a number of psychological issues as well as displace other important activities such as exercise and spending time with others. These downsides are real, and we have increasing evidence to suggest they are significant, but of course they don't apply to everyone, and using social media does not automatically guarantee that your mental health will suffer. Social media can also have some beneficial impacts, which are important to note, as we tend to focus far more on the doom and gloom.

If any of the issues raised in this chapter feel like they connect with you in some way, please reach out to someone who can help. While I hope these words prove insightful, they cannot substitute for professional guidance and treatment.

7

HOW ARE WE CHANGING THE WORLD OF FOOD BRANDS?

B rands are riding the wave of social media marketing. Surveys show that 73% of marketers believe that their efforts through social media marketing have been at least somewhat effective for their business. Through social media, brands have new ways to connect with consumers more directly. Rather than paying for an advert you hope will reach the right people, you can now target consumers directly through paid adverts on social media or, more organically, simply by creating an account and inviting consumers to like and follow.

Many brands are now using this strategy. Some kind of social platform is now used by 81% of all small and medium businesses, while 91% of retail brands use two or more social media channels. There are now over 25 million brand accounts on Instagram, with 80% of users following at least one. If a brand is not using social media influencer marketing as a strategy to better attract its target audience, now would be a good time for them to re-evaluate and consider it, because it's not going away any time soon.

The idea here is that brands can use social media to manage their online presence and make sure they keep in touch with their audience directly. This includes responding to comments, mentions and messages. Almost three-quarters (71%) of consumers who have had a positive experience with a brand on social media are likely to recommend the brand to their friends and family. On top of that, influencer marketing is becoming the primary method used to find new online customers, as well as building awareness of a brand and its products.

Food brands thrive on social media

Lauren Armes is the CEO and founder of Welltodo, as well as a business coach to wellness entrepreneurs. She identifies the appeal of social media marketing: "I work with a high volume of entrepreneurs, coaching and mentoring them on how to commercialise a passion for wellness. Social media is an obvious channel for promoting any business proposition and reaching an incredibly engaged audience – and wellness seems to be a bit of a sweet spot for social media because it often comes with beautiful, aesthetically appealing imagery of both the product/ service and the 'ideal' consumer."

But how essential is social media to building and maintaining a successful business in the world of food? Fab Giovanetti, a marketing consultant and founder of the Creative Impact Co, says: "As a marketer I see [social media] as a marketing tool that helps you create the right content for your audience, just like PR or a blog may be. I do not believe all social is for everyone, and I always help my clients think about their own preferences and where their audience lives. Ideally, social media should be leading to better conversation, rather than just engagement. Let's be honest, a business that does not sell is not really IN business."

Lauren Armes agrees: "A food brand which is designed to appeal to an individual who, let's say, values sustainability, health and advocates fun and freedom, is in a position to reach that specific audience with pinpoint accuracy via social media. Data is now more lucrative than oil in the global economy, meaning any brand wanting to scale and have a significant impact, really needs to tap into these channels."

There's no doubt that social media makes it far easier and cheaper to reach your target audience. You no longer need to rely on incredibly expensive advertisements on television or in magazines, which can be completely out of the reach of most start-ups and small businesses. Social media is free to join, and while brands can choose to pay for promoted posts on the apps, they don't have to.

A more recent change in the way brands advertise and promote their products and services is by using influencers. These can be micro-influencers with a few hundred or a few thousand followers, or big names on Instagram with sometimes millions of dedicated fans. When done well, influencer marketing campaigns earn about $6.50 for each dollar spent, so they're well worth the investment.

Back to Lauren Armes: "In some ways, it can be hugely beneficial for a brand to align itself with an expert or individual with credibility and influence over the brand's target audience. Consumers increasingly want to understand both the story behind a brand (which can often see the founder themselves

become a person of influence) and have their purchasing decisions validated by somebody who they trust. Via social media, a
one-way portal into one individual's world can have a profound
impact on the decisions that audience member makes – be it
what they eat, wear or where they go. The benefits, therefore,
of a food business working with a social media influencer who
genuinely endorses the product can be immense."

When brands work with influencers, they can get great content that they can use for their own social media, reach their
target audience when the influencer posts sponsored content on
their own page, and give customers ideas for how to use their
products, particularly if the influencer creates recipes.

Fab Giovanetti again: "Overall, I believe influencers are just
one type of advocate you can tap into. However, they have a more
effective way to get their audiences to act and purchase than your
average customer since people would look to them for recommendations on specific products."

Having a platform on social media comes with a certain
responsibility, and a good influencer will recognise this and take
it seriously.

I have my own experience of working with brands on social
media. I don't do it so much any more – mainly because I tend to be
approached by health-focused brands and I refuse to say anything
incorrect or illegal (more on that later) – but I've spoken to a few
amazing people who do work with brands and asked them about
their experiences: Becky Excell, gluten-free blogger @beckyexcell;
Izy Hossack, food blogger and Instagrammer @izyhossack; and
Sara Kiyo Popowa, the artist behind @shisodelicious.

Becky has a following across Instagram, Twitter, Facebook
and YouTube. She told me: "I've worked with brands on a regular

basis over many years now. It's an incredibly important part of what I do purely because it's allowed me to turn my blog, my social channels and my content creation into my full-time job. Being able to work on my blog full time has meant that I'm able to create more recipes, travel to more places to create guides, and generally just continue to make people's lives easier. It's been very natural working with brands for me. Many of the brands I work with are brands I post about and buy anyway. Working with brands has allowed me to do what I love for a living, it's made me happy and that's the most important thing in life, right?"

Becoming an influencer is something a lot of people aspire to, and that usually involves building an audience large enough for brands to want to work with you. Izy says: "There are a lot of people who [become influencers] because they've seen others make money from it and they think it's a good route to get rich, so they go about it totally the wrong way, which gives other influencers a bad name." Is the money or the fame and popularity more of the appeal for people? "It's probably a combination of both because you get invited to events and meet other people who are popular or famous, and you get to go on press trips, all while making money. So, it's probably a combination of both that attracts people to it." The external validation from social media certainly can't hurt either. Sara says: "I feel a strong responsibility towards my followers and how my public choices will be perceived. I say no to most brand offers I get. Many products come in plastic wrapping, or have ingredients or elements that are so obviously non-carbon footprint friendly. Since doing #threemonthsofminimalplastic (started January [2019] and ongoing) I have been unable to take many offers based on that. For the brands that appear on my social, many tend to be friends (paid or unpaid coverage), or part of a support network where I know that there's a mutual support that's not based on money."

How does Becky navigate working with brands with authenticity? "It's been really straightforward for me. The recipes I create and the products I talk about are always gluten-free, so I always work with brands that are gluten-free too. You would never see me working with a food brand's product that contains gluten – I mean, I have to eat gluten-free so it wouldn't work! When I work with brands, I always ensure I have a lot of creative freedom so that I can make the content relevant to my audience and something they would be interested in – just like they are with my non-branded content."

Izy navigates this responsibility by just not talking about health and instead focusing on what she does best: "I make food because it tastes good. I don't put labels on what I eat, and I've never said I have any dietary restrictions, I don't want people to think about that when it comes to me, I just want people to think I make nice food."

There's a misconception that working with social media influencers always involves them posting on their social media channels as a kind of advertisement, but for many influencers this is just a small part of what they do, and they see their pages as more of a portfolio. Sara, for example, is an incredible photographer. "I prefer 'off-public' work to be honest, photography and consulting clients where the work I do will be used by the client but not shared on my social." Izy also does this kind of work, as well as running photography workshops for other bloggers who are keen to up their game. Her Instagram is a portfolio of her work, which shows potential clients how good she is and what they could learn.

Brands make mistakes online too

Of course, while social media can be an amazing tool, there's no clear manual for starting a food brand or becoming an influencer, and mistakes do happen.

"Social media, for any business, must form part of an integrated marketing strategy – and my feeling is that it's not always the best tool for every business," says Lauren Armes. "I encourage entrepreneurs that I work with to see it as a means of engaging authentically with their target consumer – enabling meaningful conversations that might create a feedback loop that improves the product or service. A way of cultivating and connecting with customers so that there is a clear return on investment. I also encourage them to avoid creating content for content's sake and instead, use social media as a communication tool – which amplifies a clear business mission and creates credible, meaningful, genuine relationships with customers."

Fah sees this too. She has identified two interlinked mistakes brands make: "The first one is brands shouting rather than conversing on social. Social media should be mainly about listening, reacting and educating (or inspiring). This leads me to my second mistake: brands are not as good as influencers at telling stories, and stories are the most powerful tool we have to connect with people. Fewer product shots, more stories."

Some brands have taken this idea of storytelling and run with it, aligning the brand with the story of the founder, who then becomes an influencer themselves (if they weren't already one before).

"A lot of brands will understand that the point of using a creator is that they know their audience and can create content that both the brand and the audience will like," Izy explains.

"Some brands, however, are still stuck in the idea that they're buying advertising space where you're just the photographer, and they want you to write a caption that includes their key phrases and has their product in the shot in a very unnatural way. You just have to deal with it and explain to them how you work."

It's interesting how some brands really understand the influencer world, whereas others are still stuck in the past. Sometimes brands will ask creators to post a specific image the brand has created, not realising that if that's what they want they simply need to create an advertisement or post it on their own page and turn it into a promoted post. An influencer isn't simply an advertising space, they do something a bit different.

Despite being super-successful, Izy still regularly gets asked to work in exchange for products or exposure. To which she replies "people die of exposure".

Death by exposure aside, the idea Lauren presents of 'content for content's sake' is an interesting one, as I've often heard that the limiting factor for any brand on social media isn't usually time or money, it's the content itself. There is a pressure to post on a regular, even daily, basis in order to not fall behind, which can dilute the messages a brand wants to get across. It can also lead to them forming unsuitable partnerships with influencers.

Dodgy influencer campaigns

Influencer marketing is big business now, and when brands feel the pressure to create huge amounts of content, or don't understand the rules and regulations, it can be risky and frustrating for both parties.

Izy commented: "I have to be very picky in terms of the brands I work with, because I get quite a lot of offers for sponsored content. Working with what the PR wants, what the brand wants, delivering everything in a really short timeframe... all of these things are stressful enough on their own. I also have to consider if the brand fits with what I buy myself and use, and what would fit on my Instagram. It's hard to choose, but I'm very picky with who I work with and what I'm willing to do. I don't work with brands that I would never use myself, and obviously I never lie in my captions, even if it's what I've been told to say. For example, a maple syrup brand wanted me to talk about how their product is lower in sugar than sugar itself, and I just refused to say that because I don't agree with this at all."

Izy's right about that. Maple syrup is definitely still sugar. Just like... white sugar, but in liquid form. This is one of the biggest issues with influencer marketing: misleading or even illegal health claims.

Lauren recognises this too. "There are obviously opportunities to partner with social media influencers which do not prove fruitful – an example might be where a brand seeks endorsement from an influencer who is not aligned with the brand's values and contradicts these values in some way. Another mistake might be where a brand's proposition requires trust and credibility from its audience but this is not conveyed through credible content. Credible content, in this case, might be endorsed by an expert, backed by evidence, or scientifically proven. Food brands can often fall foul of the rule book by making health claims that aren't justified, proven, or legally allowed, and in some way mislead the consumer as to their efficacy or expected results."

Get ready, because we're about to dive into the illegal side of influencing.

There is an EU Register on nutrition and health claims which lists all the 256 approved health claims that are permitted for use in the UK. That's right, there are only 256 approved claims that can be made about the relationship between food and health. For example, a health claim would be something like 'vitamin A is required for normal functioning of the immune system'.

Health claims are useful because they provide information to consumers, they aid consumer choice, and they can be used as a marketing tool to increase sales. However, they can also be misleading and incorrect. For example, you can't claim or imply that food can treat, prevent or cure any disease or medical condition. Because food isn't medicine.

Let's take the example of oats.

Nutrient: Beta-glucans (found in oats).
Claim: 'Beta-glucans contribute to the maintenance of normal blood cholesterol levels.'
Conditions: 'The claim may be used only for food which contains at least 1 gram of beta-glucans from oats, oat bran, barley, barley bran or from mixtures of these sources per quantified portion.'

Or, how about the example of iron:

Nutrient: Iron.
Claim: 'Iron contributes to the reduction of tiredness and fatigue.'
Conditions: 'May be used only for food which is at least

a source of iron' that is, at least 15% of the reference nutrient intake* per serving.

Importantly, reference to general, non-specific benefits of the nutrient or food for overall good health or health-related well-being may only be made if accompanied by a specific health claim. Going back to the example of oats: 'Super healthy oaty goodness!' would not be approved as it only includes a very general claim of 'goodness' – what's 'good' about it? They need to tell us. 'Full of oaty goodness – contains beta-glucans that contribute to the maintenance of normal blood cholesterol levels' includes the general claim followed by the specific health claim, so that would be approved for use on packaging and in marketing materials.

Have a look at the packaging of food products that make these claims and see if you can spot them. Big multinational corporations are usually very good at adhering to this, so have a look on the packet, or keep an eye out for the small print next time you see an advert.

You could argue that it's the responsibility of the brand to get this right and to advise influencers, and I would agree with you. When I've done work with big brands in the past they have been extremely strict about what I can and cannot say on social media to ensure they stay within the legal limits. They have teams of lawyers and experts who ensure everything is above board. Small businesses and start-ups, on the other hand, are sometimes either unaware of the list of approved health claims, or deliberately exploit the ignorance of influencers.

---

* The reference nutrient intake (RNI) is defined as the amount of a nutrient that is enough to ensure that the needs of nearly everyone (97.5%) are being met.

Keep it (il)legal

Recently, there have been a growing number of cases where the Advertising Standards Authority (ASA) has ruled that influencers are making unapproved health claims in their posts. The ASA is the UK's independent regulator of advertising across all media, and it has the power to remove entire advertising campaigns that infringe legislation.

When we suspect someone has broken the rules, any individual can report the brand and/or influencer making the claim to the ASA. The authority will investigate, ask some questions, and aim to resolve the matter informally if possible (although the complaint will still appear on the ASA website for the sake of transparency). If the matter can't be resolved informally, or it's deemed necessary, the ASA will conduct a formal investigation. It will either rule that the complaint is upheld, in which case the claim has to be removed, or not, in which case the brand or influencer is free to keep the post up as is. All rulings are published on the ASA website in public domain for everyone to see.

Some great examples of rulings on unapproved claims I've found on the ASA website include: 'Boosts metabolism', 'fat-burning', 'twice as much vitamin C as an orange', 'detox', and 'carb-blocker'.

Protein World has had a lot of shit from the public over the last few years. There was the 'Are you beach body ready?' poster which featured a thin woman and the company's weight loss collection. The campaign sparked outrage in both the UK and the US, and rightly so. Sadly, it was not banned, despite over 200 complaints to the ASA and an online petition calling for its removal that attracted more than 70,000 signatures. It was a terrible message, a play on people's insecurities, and incredibly objectifying. To be clear: all bodies are beach body ready.

This isn't the example I want to discuss, though – as you may have already observed this campaign was primarily offline. In May 2017, television personality Holly Hagan tweeted: "Always take my @ProteinWorld Carb Blockers Before a Cheat meal, contain [sic] natural ingredients and stop any unused sugars being used as fat #ad". The tweet also included a photo of Holly holding a burger with a jar of Carb Blocker pills in the shot. Two days later, Protein World posted a picture on its Instagram of a model holding a burger with chips as well as the Carb Blockers, with the caption: "We are already planning our weekend treat at PW head quarters [sic] with carb blockers at the ready! Take 2 carb blockers 30 mins before a high carb meal to stop unused sugars being stored as fat in the body! Guilt free Treat...what a dream. Shop online proteinworld.com #proteinworld #lifestyle #cheatmeal #burger". Two complaints were made, challenging whether these Carb Blockers could actually prevent unused sugars from being converted into fat and stored in the body.

There are currently just two authorised health claims on the EU Register for chromium (which was the only micronutrient Protein World could have made a claim for): 'Chromium contributes to normal macronutrient metabolism'; and 'Chromium contributes to the maintenance of normal blood glucose levels'. The claims are only allowed when foods are at least a source of trivalent chromium (15% of RNI).

The ASA ruling was as follows: "We considered that in the context of a food supplement, consumers would consider 'Carb Blocker' to refer to something that offered significantly greater prevention than the body could naturally achieve without its use, i.e. the significantly improved ability to prevent the storage of unused sugars as fat... Protein World did not provide evidence that demonstrated their product contained sufficient quantities of trivalent chromium to meet the conditions of use associated with either of the authorised health claims."

In other words, there wasn't enough chromium in the products for Protein World to be allowed the use of the health claims. Not only that, but the ASA ruled that the phrasing Protein World was using far exaggerated the actual reality of the claims of what chromium can do. The authority's ruling stated, "We told Protein World not to make health claims for foods if they were not listed as authorised in the EU Register. In particular, they must not use the product name 'Carb Blocker' or claims such as 'stop any unused sugars being stored as fat' in their advertising."

I want to be clear: this was taken down because of two complaints. Two people decided they smelled bullshit and that was enough to prevent Protein World making this ridiculously incorrect claim. So yes, your voice really does make a difference.

The new guidelines

In June 2019 the ASA partnered with television channel ITV to release a 'cheat sheet' for the stars of *Love Island*,* informing them how to make it clear when social media posts are advertisements. They clearly state that influencers have to use #ad at the start

---

* If you're not familiar with this show I'm impressed! It's everywhere...

of their posts to make it clear and transparent to their followers that the post is sponsored. Paid partnerships, gifted products and experiences, and discount codes with affiliate links all apply and all have to be declared. The guidelines state that: "Consumers shouldn't have to play detective in working out when what they see, hear or interact with is a commercial message." The ASA makes it clear that there's nothing wrong with being paid to post, as long as it's clear, which I think is a very fair message.

Social media influencers are, most of the time, not qualified experts in food and health, and so are usually unaware of the legal limits of the claims they're permitted to make. This can easily contribute to the spread of misinformation and exaggeration in terms of what a food or supplement is actually able to do. While so far many have been able to get away with it, the ASA has promised greater crackdowns on influencer posts. I can only hope they mean it.

When brands exploit influencers

Being an influencer and working with brands sounds exciting and glamorous. In fact, many children now say they want to be a social media influencer when they grow up. I remember the first few times I was gifted products by a brand – it was so exciting! I felt as if I'd 'made it'. At first, I would accept these gifts in exchange for posts so the brand would get exposure, until a marketing consultant told me I should really be charging brands for the pleasure of being publicly recommended by me. I worked with some lovely and friendly brands back in the day, but, on reflection, some of them definitely exploited me.

One superfood company I worked with (don't judge me, I know better now!) approached a number of young health bloggers to collaborate. We all found this incredibly exciting, and would receive plenty of free products (these powders were seriously expensive), be invited to exclusive events, and have affiliate links. The founders lived in London, and at one point they even invited a few of us over for dinner. With hindsight, it was a little creepy that this couple thought it was a good idea to invite a bunch of 19- and 20-year-old girls to their home. They made us feel special and pressured us to keep posting about them for free and stay loyal by not mentioning any other brands. We gave them free exposure long after we'd all started charging everyone else. We were young and impressionable, and they took advantage of that, grooming us to be their shiny little ambassadors. When I eventually told them I wasn't interested in receiving their latest product and promoting it, politely mentioning that I didn't agree with some of their marketing tactics (read: illegal claims and blog posts by dentists saying if you're really healthy you don't need to brush your teeth because our ancestors didn't), the founders instantly became aggressive, saying I was selling out to 'Big Food' and supermarkets by not supporting them, and how dare I turn my back on them after everything they had done for me. It was incredibly rude and unprofessional.

The glamorisation of influencing, and the power imbalance between brands and influencers can lead to young people being exploited. It happened to me, and to several of my friends on social media around the same time.

This power balance can also shift the other way, with influencers potentially having enough power to boycott unethical brands. Has this happened yet? As far as I know, not really. There have been many occasions where I've replied to emails from brands asking them to provide evidence for their claims, to which they either respond with YouTube links (not evidence) or don't respond at all. Now, I simply report them to the ASA. I'd encourage you to do the same.

How influential are these influencers really?

Ultimately, the role of the influencer is to build awareness around a new product, especially if it requires some explanation of how to use it or how it tastes, or even just to provide recipe inspiration.

Naturally, this then influences our food choice. If advertising didn't work, companies wouldn't spend huge amounts of money on it. The very name 'influencer' implies that the individual is influencing people to make certain decisions, nudging them in the direction of certain ideas, behaviours or actions – including deciding which kind of food to buy.

Influencer marketing is more significant here than regular advertising. Age restrictions mean that young children don't really use social media sites like Facebook or Instagram, but there's a significant children's market on YouTube.

Research with adults shows that a disclosure of an advert can counter the persuasive effects of advertising and brand attention, by activating persuasion knowledge and mitigating persuasion. In other words, when we know something is an advert we're more likely to think critically and are less likely to be influenced by it. But this is not the case for children; they can't tell the difference. For children, you need a lot more than just disclosure. They need to be aware of the fact it's an advert, sure, but they also need to understand the persuasive intent of the advert and have both the ability and motivation to resist persuasion. If advertising disclosures on vlogs, for example, are transparent about the nature of the partnership, then this won't make any difference unless the children are motivated to do something about it.

Concerns have been raised over the potential for digital marketing to be even more impactful on eating behaviour than traditional forms of exposure. Children are able to recognise adverts on television from a relatively young age due to the clear break from the programme they're watching, but in digital marketing this distinction is blurred. In order to support children to discern what digital content is actually marketing, current self-regulatory codes in the UK require that influencer marketing should be labelled with an advertising disclosure. At the very least, they have to include #AD or 'AD' in the YouTube video title.

Exposure to celebrity endorsement of high fat, salt and sugar (HFSS) foods in television commercials has been shown to increase children's preference for these products, so they ask their parents to buy these foods and end up eating more of them. Research shows that when children consume a greater quantity of snack food following food advertising exposure, either via television or the Internet, they don't compensate for this additional intake by eating a bit less at their next meal. Over time this can lead to unexpected weight gain.

Children also report viewing influencers to be more trustworthy than traditional celebrities, possibly because of increased feelings of familiarity, so you would think that children would also respond to their favourite vloggers eating these foods in the same way – and you'd be correct. When children are exposed to influencer marketing of unhealthy snacks, they eat more compared to children who are exposed to healthy food or non-food marketing. When children see influencers eating healthier snacks such as fruit, for example, they do also respond, but less strongly than to so-called 'junk' foods.

Social media influencers promote brands through their personal lives, because their aspirational lives are essentially their own personal brand. This makes them more relatable to the average consumer; we feel they're just 'one of us'. Influencers truly serve as the ultimate connection between a brand and a consumer. While we can perhaps understand that celebrities are paid to say what the brand wants, we feel that influencers are more open and candid, which gives them more credibility. This is what makes the influencer phenomenon so successful. Whereas traditional marketing targeted mostly mass audiences indiscriminately, influencers have the unique ability to target niche audiences that, until now, have often been unreachable.

Influencers are the leaders, and provide an example for those who, literally, 'follow' them. By viewing their behaviour and their preferences we're more likely to adopt those ideas for ourselves. Companies are taking advantage of this, anticipating that the positive experience and connection consumers have with an influencer is transferred to the brand by association. This electronic word of mouth is known to be incredibly credible and trusted, and successful social media influencers are masters of this.

Before the rise of social media influencers, advertising to brand consumers was very much one-sided – a consumer would only

see a product through print advertisements, posters, sponsor-
ship, or radio and television commercials, which are forced upon
us. Today, consumers can interact with a product through social
media. Watching an influencer we trust using or recommending
a product allows us to feel we're making a more informed decision
about buying it. It feels more like a choice. It is clear that social
media influencer marketing has changed the way brands interact
with consumers in a positive way, by allowing communication
to be two-way. These tactics help to explain why social media
influencer marketing is one of the biggest trends of recent years.

In the future

Where do you see the relationship between social media and the
food industry heading in the future? Lauren Armes has some
ideas: "My view is that greater regulation is required and that
where systematic regulation fails the consumer, that the consumer will put adequate pressure on brands such that they take
responsibility for their own marketing messages. The consumer is
increasingly savvy and less tolerant of brands that try to 'pull the
wool over their eyes'. In an age of 'woke washing' – where brands
leverage a cause for commercial gain – consumers demand
greater transparency, deeper evidence of brand purpose being
fulfilled, and expect that brands will walk their talk. Social media
will continue to be a powerful connection tool between brand
and consumer – but successful outcomes will rely on well thought
out, sustainable communication strategies."

   Fab Giovanetti also says she sees "experts turning into influencers", and while I agree this could be a great idea in theory,

in practice I've noticed a frightening number of qualified health-care professionals go down the Dr. Oz route – unethical but get-ting rich.

I don't see influencers going away anytime soon, and I don't want to paint a picture of immoral behaviour designed to try and make us all unwell, because that's just not true. The majority of online influencers are women, and seeing women take charge of their careers and doing something they love is a wonderful thing, and if they stopped marketing unethical products like detox teas, that would be even better.

Thankfully, Instagram has recently launched a new policy to restrict posts that encourage users to buy 'laxative' diet teas, shakes and lollipops, designed to stop under-18-year-olds from being exposed to these ineffective and harmful products. Insta-gram will allow users to report a post on the app if they believe it violates this policy. Instagram will then review the content, and if it does encourage weight-loss products the post will be restricted. When you look at these detox tea Instagram pages now, many of the squares on the grid are greyed out, and you have to confirm that you're over 18 to be able to view the post. When the content makes a miraculous claim about certain diet or weight-loss products, and is linked to an offer such as a dis-count code, it will no longer be allowed and will be removed from Instagram. Hopefully, this will mean fewer celebrities posing with appetite-suppressant lollipops and detox teas, claiming that these products are responsible for their weight loss when the whole world knows they've had surgery.

Progress!

8

HOW ARE WE CHANGING THE WORLD OF RESTAURANTS?

People want to show off and to share their experiences of eating great food, which is why most people who post food pictures do so while still at the dinner table. Some restaurants and cafes are taking advantage of this.

One of the reasons we share food pictures online is for status. Yes, we share pictures of food that we made and we're proud of as a showcase of our abilities, but we're also far more likely to post a food picture from an expensive Michelin-starred restaurant, or an exclusive food event, than we are from the local pub. These pictures make our lives look exciting and desirable.

People will tweet about the food they're craving, particularly which restaurants they're pining for. In fact, people are now more likely to tweet about craving a Nando's than they are about simply 'craving chicken' – to the point where Nando's has created an ad campaign around this. More than half of UK Twitter users log on when they're in a restaurant, any restaurant, and, of those, 37% have posted a picture of their meal.

But not only are we using the photo-sharing social networks to document what we're eating, we're using them to decide where to eat too. Nearly three-quarters of customers have used Facebook to make restaurant decisions, based on comments and images that have been shared by other users. According to research by the restaurant chain Zizzi, 30% of millennials would avoid a restaurant with a weak Instagram presence. It's now normal to sit down in a restaurant having already decided what you're going to order because you've taken the time to Google the menu and snoop around on Instagram in advance.

But it should be a two-way communication, and restaurants are rewarded for responding to customers on social media: 71% of customers say they're more likely to recommend a company that responds quickly and kindly to them on social media.

When I go on holiday somewhere, I ask my Instagram followers where I should eat, and collect their responses. I check online to see if any of the places mentioned have a social media presence, not because it's the be-all-and-end-all, but because I like seeing what kind of things they have on the menu. In some cities, like London, you'll find almost every restaurant has at least one social media account. In other places, many parts of Italy, for instance, Instagram won't help as the best places are the family-owned establishments that mainly care about enticing people as they walk past.

Picture perfect?

If a particular dish is receiving a lot of attention on Instagram, and many people are posting pictures of it, that coverage entices future customers as they want to try what's popular, and it tells the restaurant they're doing something right. It's free marketing. For owners of restaurant chains, keeping an eye on Instagram means they can also police what's actually going out in their restaurants and check the dishes are being presented correctly, even when they're not physically present.

Like it or not, social media, and Instagram in particular, has impacted on the world restaurant industry. Restaurants, cafes and bars now have to think more than ever about the aesthetics of their establishment, whether it's elaborate flower displays, living walls, neon light installations, or quirky bathroom tiles. And then there's the food, which has to be visually appealing enough to be considered worthy of sharing online.

I asked Izy Hossack, who has partnered with restaurants in the past, and been offered free meals, what she thinks about how social media has affected the restaurant industry. "It's a double-edged sword. I think Instagram has helped a lot of small businesses in the food industry because sharing images of food at restaurants or pop-ups or street food vans is one of the main ways they would get noticed. It's so expensive to run advertising campaigns, and if all you have to do is give a free meal to 10 influencers and get the same reach as you would from a single-page ad in a magazine, it's far more worth it cost-wise. But on the other hand, it influences the brands themselves to start making things more Instagram-friendly. So, they might design their whole restaurants around Instagram and change their menus, and then you just end up with people sitting in restaurants taking photos the whole time and not actually enjoying the food. If you make food that's amazing for Instagram and just tastes like crap... it'll have no longevity." Izy's prime concern is one I share – that influencers and social media are encouraging restaurants to make food that's aesthetically pleasing and gets the likes, but doesn't satisfy the palate.

While Facebook may have its recipe-sharing groups, Pinterest users are making everything in Mason jars, and YouTube is filled with recipe videos, Instagram is still very much the king of food sharing. When a certain dish or food item, such as freakshakes or the cronut, becomes an Instagram sensation, it results in people queuing down the street to get into the restaurant and literally snap it up. Starbucks' Unicorn Frappuccino is a classic example of something looking good for the 'gram without actually tasting good. I haven't met a single person who has tried it and wasn't disappointed by the flavour. That didn't stop people from sharing their pictures online though. There was even a phase where restaurants would put glitter in foods, for example glitter lattes – even glitter gravy. Raindrop cakes taste like nothing, galaxy doughnuts stain your fingers, charcoal ice cream turns your teeth black, sushi burritos fall apart. In the end, what these viral foods lack in flavour, they make up for in likes and comments.

It's easy to dismiss it as style over substance, but social media is an incredibly useful marketing tool for restaurants. Restaurants and bars are increasingly giving influencers a seat at the table, reaching out to them alongside critics and traditional media, even sometimes hosting events especially for them, something that would have been unthinkable at the turn of the millennium.

A case study of vegan burgers

Rachel Hugh is the co-founder of The Vurger Co., a 100% vegan fast-food brand. Vurger owes a lot of its success to social media. "When we started on our journey creating The Vurger Co., we had to overcome so many obstacles, primarily raising funding to even open the doors to a permanent restaurant site. This fundamental obstacle became the bane of our life, as no investor believed in the long-term growth of creating a restaurant business just based on vegan burgers, in fact most would call us insane. So we knew the only way to make this work would be to reach to those who are already talking about, discussing and are passionate about this way of living, this type of food and lifestyle."

This, she says, is where social media comes in. "When we had our first ever market stalls, pop-up events and festivals, literally the only outreach we would do would be on social media – primarily Instagram. This is how our customers got to know who we are, follow our journey, see our struggles, get to know our brand from the ground up. That, in today's market, is absolutely crucial to the success of the longevity of any brand and we learnt that pretty much from the start. Our super-fans became the advocates for our brand, without even asking, that's the true power of connecting with your audience."

How does she think the business would be different without social media? A lot, apparently. "Without any form of social media, I have absolutely no idea how we would have been able to reach our customers and speak to them directly. Gaining their early feedback, listening to their comments and understanding what they wanted from us as a brand was absolutely crucial to our business journey and, without social media, I truly don't believe there is another way to do that in such a dynamic way."

Social media is now having an impact on various decisions in restaurants, including menu, colour scheme and décor.

"We, along the journey, mainly have gained inspiration from reaching out to our customers, coming from a genuine place and asking them the questions that most people would be scared to do." Rachel continues, "We would ask consistently – what do they like about a particular menu item, should it be dropped from the menu, we ask where our customers want to see us opening up next, where else we could be looking at worldwide... so many business decisions are based on true, genuine customer feedback that again you wouldn't be able to get so well without some form of formal customer survey that wouldn't even target the genuine brand supporters anyway!"

Some restaurants take things a step further, even changing the décor to be more 'Instagrammable'. Grind, the popular London cafe-bar chain, went so far as to change their tables to marble in 2016 specifically because it looks good on Instagram. And, according to them, it's paid off! Aside from tabletops, they also tailor the menu according to what's Instagram-friendly, which makes sense because many people are now encountering the food via social media before they read it on a menu, so appearance does matter.

"It has taken a long time to build up our customer base, and the way we did that was through the engagement we were receiving on Instagram." Says Rachel, "As a result, our Instagram page @thevurgerco became our 'go to' hub where people would literally eat with their eyes, coming into store and asking our team to have exactly what we have posted on Instagram today."

It's not just consumers who are judging food based solely on a photo, chefs are doing it too. It's led to a growing number of chefs who are cooking for the 'gram – where someone will put a dish together without any concern for whether or not it actually tastes good, just as long as the aesthetic is right. The most important thing with any dish should surely be how it tastes. However, one aspect of building a great dish in a restaurant is now undeniably how it looks, because if it's pretty it's going to appear on Instagram and be shared potentially around the world.

This explains the rise in popularity of certain food items, like baked eggs (#yolkporn), avocado toast and freakshakes. These foods go viral and show how useful it can be to have aesthetically pleasing foods on the menu. It's all extra pressure for the chefs and owners.

Rachel at The Vurger Co. has felt this pressure too. "I think inevitably your food has to be presentable, look eye-catching, look like something most people would want, but we [at Vurger] had the added pressure of ensuring everybody felt welcome looking to a vegan food brand for inspiration. Ultimately, we share customer shots, so everything is genuinely what any customer who walks in would have in front of their eyes!"

Sharing customer photos is an incredibly effective tool for building a following online, as it taps into something I mentioned in the introduction: variable rewards, where rewards are delivered randomly (like with a slot machine). When you tag the restaurant you never know which photo you share is going to be reposted on their feed, and the anticipation that this might happen triggers a dopamine response in your brain. It's a very clever marketing tactic because we do feel like it's a reward to have our image reposted – it's an honour!

But while many chefs and restaurants love it when customers take pictures and share them online, some even heavily relying on it for marketing purposes, others are less keen. High-end chefs, such as David Chang at Michelin-starred Ko in New York, have banned diners from taking photos of food, and The Fat Duck in Berkshire, owned by Heston Blumenthal, has a no-flash policy. A group of French chefs, including one with the coveted three Michelin stars, has been threatening to ban cameras and mobile phones from their restaurants entirely. While this may seem a bit extreme, some of their criticisms are well-founded: pausing a conversation to take pictures derails it, flash photography disturbs everyone around you, and spending so much time taking pictures that your food goes cold isn't the fault of the chef. Some chefs are just fed up. Renowned French chef Michel Roux once said, "A picture on a phone cannot possibly capture the flavours."

One cafe in Sydney, Australia has a policy that states: 'No photos of the restaurant, no photos of the kitchen, no photo-shoots, no video shoots, no flash, no excessive photo taking, and please keep the aisles clear.' Guests are still allowed to take amateur pics of their food and friends, as long as the photography is confined to their personal space and doesn't disturb anyone. The owners claim they were forced to implement the rules when they noticed bloggers and influencers wandering around for their personal photoshoots, taking up valuable restaurant space without actually spending any money. I have seen this kind of thing in some London cafes that have made it onto the 'most Instagrammable' lists. It's incredibly annoying. By all means take a quick picture, but when your photographer is taking up space, spending 10 minutes getting various shots of you posing with your latte, it's a serious inconvenience to both the staff and other customers. That's the point where I start to find it uncomfortable, and is probably why I tend to avoid those kinds of places now.

Behind the scenes, Lauren Armes says that social media is helping investors decide where to put their money. "Investors are looking for a brand with a commercially scalable proposition and an opportunity for real returns. Naturally, if a brand already has a loyal, engaged following (whether in the form of an email database or a social media following) then this is of great benefit. A presence on social media is only valuable for an investor if the audience is actively purchasing the brand's product or service – it is otherwise commercially meaningless."

Overall, Rachel Hugh sees social media as being a major positive to a food business. "It's a fantastic tool to connect with your customers, showcase your brand from an authentic standpoint and build your key relationships with your super-fans by listening directly in real time with their feedback – where else can you do that? People pay marketing agencies thousands and thousands to 'build a brand persona' or 'connect with a customer base' – you can do that for yourself and, trust me, your customers will love hearing from you directly. Just speak from the heart, put in the time and keep going."

When influencers and restaurants work together

When influencers and the restaurant industry collide, it can result in something beautiful, or it can be a total mess.

Sometimes partnering with the right influencer can change

everything for the better. Early on, The Vurger Co. partnered with vegan influencer and recipe developer Gaz Oakley, of @avantegardevegan fame. In 2019, Gaz had over a million followers on YouTube and Instagram combined. This partnership turned out to be a smart move. "When we began, we wanted as much feedback as possible on our product. Gaz started his journey around the same time as us, also being from Wales, and we reached out to him to invite him to one of our first ever pop-ups to gain some feedback from some amazing people in the industry. Gaz, being the kind person that he is, came all the way to London to try our menu and offer his advice and feedback. The relationship was born from a very genuine place, and watching his platform grow and his profile become what it is today has been genuinely one of the most exciting things to see. Having both continued on the path we have, in the same space, when we finally managed to open our own restaurant, we knew it was the right time to actually get the chance to work together, and now Gaz is our official Executive Chef. So, the best things are born from social media; how else would we have known about his incredible talent and also been able to directly speak to him without the connected world we live in today?"

Alongside this incredible partnership (I've tasted the resulting food and it's damn amazing), The Vurger Co. has occasionally offered influencers to dine for free at the restaurant. This wasn't an easy decision for the team to make. "It's such a tough decision for our business as we genuinely cannot afford to give anything away for free. But we took the decision that those who have supported us from the beginning, who have genuinely spread the word about our brand, and continue to do so without demanding anything in return, should be rewarded in some way. The fact that as a small brand we are unable to provide any monetary ambassador programmes like others do, this became the best way to ensure that our super-fans could get hold of our food." While Vurger has offered some influencers to dine for free, Rachel was keen to point out that they don't coerce anyone to say anything they don't mean. "We have never told anyone what to say, we want everyone to speak their truth. We genuinely don't see this as a bad thing because everyone we interact with already loves what we do, so we never have to 'convince' someone to say something or pay people to have an opinion. That's where the lines get blurred and isn't something I would encourage ever."

So there you have it, proof that influencer–restaurant partnerships can be a good thing!

Unhappy chefs

When food brands partner with influencers, it's generally the brands who reach out, offering products in exchange for exposure. With restaurants it's often the other way around – influencers will reach out and ask for free food in exchange for exposure.

Some influencers have review blogs and do nothing but review restaurants on their social media, and I feel it makes sense for them to ask for a free meal in exchange for a review. However, some chefs are unhappy about influencers reaching out to them for free food.

On a fateful day in April 2019, Duncan Welgemoed, chef and part-owner of the restaurant Africola in Adelaide, was checking his emails when he saw a request from a contestant on the Australian reality TV cooking show *My Kitchen Rules*. She asked to dine for free in his restaurant, and in return she would post some stories on her Instagram, thereby giving him and his restaurant exposure. Except, Africola didn't need the exposure. It's one of Australia's hottest restaurants. Celebrities like Katy Perry dine there and pay for their food. And anyway, his own Instagram account had far more followers than the influencer, so really it was totally pointless for him.

He responded to the request, sharing it on his Instagram stories for all to see: "How about you do the right thing and pay for your meal, like everyone else, you do not generate any hype or actual dollars for any business you post about. The ATO [Australian Taxation Office], suppliers nor staff care about exposure. If Katy Perry can pay for a meal in my restaurant, so can you." His response went viral.

One business owner has taken this rejection of influencer culture even further. CVT Soft Serve, a popular food truck in Los Angeles, started to receive weekly requests from Instagram influencers who promised to post a photo of their ice cream in exchange for not having to pay. Nicchi, the owner, has always said no, but then he decided he had had enough, and made his feelings very publicly known. Nicchi went viral after posting a sign that read, 'influencers pay double', sharing on Instagram that he would 'never give you a free ice cream in exchange for a post'. He tagged the image with the hashtag #InfluencersAreGross, and it spread around the globe. Now Nicchi says his business is booming, attracting fans across southern California who share his disdain of influencers. By the way, his ice cream costs just $4, so it seems a bit mad to me that someone would be demanding that for free. In response to his post, he claims he has received numerous interview requests and news coverage from around the world. His customers doubled in number overnight, and he gained thousands of new followers on Instagram. I doubt many influencers have the balls to contact him now.

Frustrated chefs around the world have taken to screenshotting requests from influencers for free food and forwarding them to prominent Australian restaurant reviewer John Lethlean, who has been publishing them on his Instagram under the hashtag #couscousforcomment.* While the hashtag has been popularised by Lethlean, it was started back in 2016 by Tim Philips-Johansson, co-owner of the Sydney bar and restaurant Bulletin Place, after an influencer contacted him asking for a free meal in exchange for a favourable review. Lethlean claims he publishes these comments mainly because he's offended by the influencers' behaviour and wants people to know just how demanding and shameless they can be. It seems he is far from alone in thinking this, and his followers rejoice in making jokes at the influencers' expense.

Some chefs and restaurant owners have even said they felt blackmailed by influencers, some of whom threatened to write bad reviews unless they received free or discounted food.

While for most young people Instagram is the place to find out where to eat, sites like TripAdvisor still hold a lot of sway, especially from Gen X. On top of that, anyone can write a

---

* 'Couscous for comment' is a play on 'cash for comment' – an Australian scandal where paid advertisements on radio were presented to the audience as simply editorial commentary. The radio hosts had been paid to give favourable comment to companies without disclosure.

Facebook review, even if they've never actually been to the place or used the services. One piece of bad press or one powerful influencer can potentially cause a flurry of one-star reviews from people who, until that day, had perhaps not even heard of the place, or didn't care about it anyway.

To show just how misleading online reviews can be, one journalist created a fake restaurant on TripAdvisor – his shed in south London. The Shed in Dulwich was created with a cheap burner phone, a vague address (so there could be no walk-ins), a simple website and an air of exclusivity. It was advertised as an appointment-only restaurant where each dish is named after a mood, such as love, contemplation, comfort or happy. Over several months, the journalist asked his friends to post fake positive reviews, each one from a different device to fool the system, and gradually The Shed began to climb in the rankings. Soon, he was getting phone calls asking for bookings, which he fielded by claiming they were fully booked, and receiving CVs from people looking for jobs. Six months after its initial invention, The Shed at Dulwich – a non-existent restaurant – was listed as the number 1 restaurant in London. Eventually the page was shut down, but it's impressive they made it that far. I think the journalist succeeded at proving his point that online reviews are often an unreliable source of information and can be deceiving.

Free food

Chefs would generally agree that having a respected, experienced critic review their restaurant is an amazing thing, but a lot of young people no longer buy newspapers or magazines. Instead, they rely on social media, and if you don't engage with them online on some level you'll miss out.

I don't want this to be a shit-all-over-influencers party, but while I think there are many great influencers out there doing great things, some give the entire group a bad rep.

There are still many occasions where restaurants will partner with a PR company, and part of the marketing strategy will be to reach out to influencers to enjoy the food in exchange for posts. Personally, I receive such emails several times a month. I haven't accepted one of these invitations for a long time, because I always worry: should you post about a free meal even if you didn't enjoy it? Simply out of obligation? Some people don't care because they're happy they get free food, others are afraid of how the restaurant would react if they don't post, and others simply say, "If I don't like it, I'm not posting".

Does Izy enjoy the food more when she pays for it or when it's free? It depends, was her reply. "I was part of a brunch club, and we'd get invites to places, and because there were six of us, we'd be offered pretty much everything on the menu. So, we could share and taste everything on the menu, whereas when you pay for yourself you generally have to choose one dish – that was amazing." She adds: "I feel guilty when I go for a free meal, even if I'm posting about it. But I do always make sure to tip when I get a free meal." Very good point – any social media exposure doesn't do anything for the staff, who have to work regardless of whether you paid for a meal or not.

People often aren't clear about whether they have paid for a meal or if it's gifted. With brands, the guidelines tend to be very clear that you have to include #AD or #sponsored, but with restaurants many people don't declare any #gifted meals. For me, personally, I would prefer people to be honest and declare when they get something for free, even if it were legal to be ambiguous.

We live in an age of 'snap first, eat and drink later', and that attitude is already having a significant impact on which restaurants we choose to give our hard-earned cash. Social media is word of mouth on steroids – with a single picture you can reach and influence thousands of people. In the end, though, however pretty the dish is, the food will hopefully speak for itself. Instagram might get people in the door, but it won't keep them there.

A final word for any influencers

If you're an influencer online who is working with brands and/or restaurants, please follow the guidelines and declare everything, using #AD and #gifted. Transparency is so important for building trust online. Make sure you're only using legal and approved health claims, which you can find online, or ask a registered nutritionist or dietitian for help. Or if that's not available, ask the brand to back up their health claims. They should easily be able to do this if it's something they've considered and researched.

9

FOOD BLOGS AND CULINARY PLAGIARISM

There are millions and millions of food blogs out there, and every recipe online now has social media icons that encourage you to share it with friends to spread the word. While I don't see blogs as a form of social media in the same way as Instagram or Pinterest, there's no denying that there's a strong link between them. Blogs have had a considerable impact on the food landscape and their impact is worth delving into.

The most obvious example of a famous food blog has to be that of Julie Powell, who was immortalised in the 2009 film *Julie & Julia*. The story, for those of you who aren't familiar or would like a reminder, goes like this: in 2002, a 30-year-old secretary from New York decided to add some spice to her life (pun intended) by spending one year cooking all 524 recipes in the 1961 classic *Mastering the Art of French Cooking* by the legendary Julia Child, Louisette Bertholle and Simone Beck.

Rather than simply do this quietly for herself, Julie Powell started a blog, called 'The Julie/Julia Project' where she wrote about all the recipes and her thoughts throughout the year. At first, no one really read it except her friends, but then the audience started to grow, particularly after her blog was featured in an article in *The New York Times*. On the back of this, she was offered a book deal. *Julie and Julia: 365 Days, 524 Recipes, 1 Tiny Apartment Kitchen* was published in 2006. Julie wasn't offered a book deal because she was an incredible writer, it was down to the fact that she had an established audience who read her blog. Her publishers knew that a market for the book already existed, which would make the book far easier to sell.

It's important to note that this book wasn't a cookbook, it was a memoir. It would take a few more years before food bloggers would be asked to write recipe books.

Before bloggers became cookbook authors, they were (and still are) sharing their recipes online, including on social media. Bloggers often use social media as a way to drive traffic to blogs, by sharing images, teasers and links to recipes. Almost immediately, the rising popularity of social media brought with it a growing problem: people stealing and plagiarising recipes.

Izy Hossack is the blogger behind Top with Cinnamon and has over 200,000 followers on her Instagram account @izyhossack. She has also had plenty of experience of others stealing her recipes. "A lot of people are scalping content from blogs because they use it to build traffic on their own websites. This often happens with recipes that do well on Pinterest – people will steal popular recipes from Pinterest and repost them on their website, so they get the traffic instead."

But people don't just steal content to post on blogs, they also do it on Instagram. "It happens a lot on Instagram where people will reuse an image of mine, and sometimes they tag and credit me, other times they don't. Technically they should be paying for usage." But according to Izy, most bloggers don't mind if they are tagged as it will hopefully drive traffic back to their Instagram page and therefore back to their website.

You can download repost apps that let you repost images and entire captions from other Instagram accounts, which happens to my images on a regular basis. What I like about these apps is that both the image and the caption have my Instagram handle very visible, so it's clear where the credit lies. So, it doesn't bother me personally when people do this as it's so clearly marked as my creation.

It's not just individuals who will do this, though; sometimes brands do it too. Izy again: "I recently had a brand – a bulk food shop in London – who had regrammed some of my photos a few times, which they hadn't asked permission for, but I was OK with it because they had tagged me [in the image]. But then later they reposted an image and, in the caption, had copied and pasted the entire recipe from my blog. The point is, they're allowed to repost the image because then if someone wants to make the recipe they have to go through to my blog to find it, which means I receive some ad revenue, and maybe that person spends some time exploring other recipes on there. But when they steal the recipe like that, what benefit am I getting from that? Nothing."

How does Izy navigate that scenario? "Whenever that happens, I write a comment on the post informing them that I haven't given them permission to use this, that it's my copyright, and ask them to take it down. Most of the time they do." What does she do if they don't? "You can report it on Instagram and Pinterest that someone has stolen your content. With that you have to provide examples of where your image is from, so you have to provide the source."

Pinterest is apparently really good at taking down stolen content, and usually do it within 24-48 hours. They even send you an email informing you when it's done. Instagram, however, isn't so great at dealing with this problem, and takes a lot longer to remove stolen content from the app.

Understandably, when someone steals your content it doesn't feel great. "It's shit, because it shows they don't respect you at all," complains Izy. "The bare minimum someone has to do is link back to a recipe they've adapted or ask to repost your photo. And yet some people can't even do that; they just take content and pretend it's theirs. Sometimes people have even stolen my content and used it as sponsored content on their own websites. They're literally getting paid for this post, and yet they couldn't even link back and say it was adapted from my recipe?"

There is a term for the stealing and reusing of recipes and passing them off as your own - culinary plagiarism. Although this term is more commonly used to describe chefs who copy dishes from other restaurants, right down to how it's plated up and served, it is now also being applied to the online world. The Internet has made plagiarism much easier than it was in the past. Where before we'd have to eat or work at a restaurant to know what the food is like, now we can just type something into Google or search the hashtag on Instagram and see hundreds of images we can copy.

It's amazing how little respect people can have for online content. We think that because we can find it and save it so easily, that we then also have the right to use it for our own purposes. We confuse what is publicly visible (almost everything on the Internet) with what is in the public domain. This is especially true for images.

Music is far easier to protect. On YouTube any breach of copyright is automatically detected, a warning notice appears, and the sound is removed from the offending video. Images are much harder to track. Part of the problem is a lack of awareness: people don't know that these images belong to someone and assume they're free because they're right there and free to view. But even when people are aware, there's still often a lack of respect and a sense of entitlement. We think that the Internet is such a large place, it's unlikely anyone will ever find out we stole their image. And even if they do find it, what's the biggest repercussion? You'll be asked to take it down. That's usually it. Particularly when it comes to bloggers, you're not going to take someone to court over one image, it's not worth it. So, there isn't really any incentive for people to respect someone else's intellectual property here, apart from being a decent human being, of course.

There are some things bloggers can do to protect their images, although they aren't perfect. Izy has some of these in place. "You can use watermarks, which are harder to remove so people can't simply lift the images and repost them elsewhere. You can also have an alert system set up with Google alerts so you can see if your name has been used somewhere and see if they've copied your recipe without asking. Other than that, there's not really much you can do, unfortunately."

Kind of depressing, really.

From blog to book

Izy is an example of someone who has been able to convert her food blog into a book deal – her book *The Savvy Cook* has some of my favourite recipes in it.* What I found interesting is that, while Izy gave many examples where someone had stolen her online recipes, the same couldn't be said for those from the book. "I've occasionally seen people post a recipe from a book as an extract, where they share which book the recipe has come from. I feel that if people are cooking from a cookbook then they're more likely to respect it as they've paid money for it." It also hopefully means that if readers like the recipe they'll consider buying her book too.

The difference in the way people treat online recipes compared to cookbook recipes is astounding. I think there are a number of reasons for this. First is the fact that, as soon as people pay money for something and physically hold it in their hands, it has more worth in their eyes. In addition, books have been around for far longer than the Internet, and book etiquette is more normalised and accepted in society – we know copying and pasting from another book isn't OK. The beauty of the online world is that anyone with an Internet connection can start a blog. There are millions of recipe blogs out there, but the marker of a successful recipe blog is to take it offline. Of course, this isn't always true, but our attitude towards a blog changes massively when there's a physical book to accompany it. I experienced this first-hand with my own family. My parents didn't really understand 'this social media thing', but as soon as I signed a contract with a publisher it completely changed how they viewed my work. After all, while anyone can start a blog, not everyone gets a book

---

* *The Savvy Cook* (2017) has a recipe for a vegetarian 'chorizo' dip that is honestly life-changing. I never tell people the ingredients before they taste it, and not one person has ever been able to tell that there's no chorizo in it. They're all shocked. That's how good it is.

deal. Blogs are common, books far less so. And when something is rarer, we again see it as more valuable.

Izy had been blogging for about two years when she was contacted by a publisher and asked to write a book. When she first started blogging, she had no idea where it was going to go, but then "After a while I started seeing other bloggers getting book deals, mainly in the US, so I figured we were about four years behind here in the UK. I did want to write a book, but that only became a goal further down the line; I didn't expect it or aim for it right from the start."

"I think having a book legitimises [the blogging]. It's crazy to think that someone could just pick this up in a shop. It's also terrifying as online you have your audience who know and enjoy your blog otherwise they wouldn't be there, whereas when a book goes out to the public anyone can find it and leave a bad review if they're not a fan." There's a big difference between someone commenting 'that looks delicious!' under a blog post, and spending money on a book.

Back when Izy's first book was published, it wasn't at all common for bloggers in the UK to get publishing deals. Now, it's still not something that's handed out to everyone, but it's become more normal for bloggers and Instagrammers. "In the US, it's very common for publishers to approach a blogger with a specific topic in mind, as they know it'll be cheaper (food bloggers will usually both develop and photograph the recipes), and they can get away with paying them a lot less as they often don't have agents or experience with books. I think this can give bloggers a bad name, as the books aren't always that amazing."

Bloggers who get book deals usually include some of their 'greatest hits' from the blog as part of the collection, which serves as a way for them to link back to their online roots and connect the online to the offline in some way. In fact, they are often encouraged to do so by the publisher themselves.

In the UK, there's been a big rise in fitness bloggers writing either recipe books, or lifestyle books that feature both exercises and recipes. What generally separates these books from those written by food bloggers is that the publisher has to bring in a team of people to shoot, style and edit the images. The blogger creates the recipes, but that's pretty much it. With books by celebrities there's usually a ghostwriter who helps develop the recipes, but fitness bloggers are given free reign and it's up to the in-house team to make it work. To be quite frank, so many of these books are awfully written with terrible recipes that either don't work or don't taste good. I have heard horror stories from food stylists who follow the recipe and simply cannot get the promised result, and so have to modify and improvise just to create something that can be photographed in time. These are bloggers who have been given book deals because of their popularity, not because of their cooking skills. They usually sell well, though, there's no denying that. I've been gifted many such books over the years, and I don't think I've made an enjoyable recipe from any of them.

How does the copyright thing work?

As soon as you create a piece of content, whether it's an image, a song, a short story, or an essay, you automatically own the copyright. In other words: you don't have to have it formally copyrighted, it's instantly your intellectual property. This means no one else can use it unless you assign them the copyright, usually in exchange for a fee.

In Izy's case it works like this. "As a photographer you usually create a set of images for a brand and they pay you for your time – the time it takes to create those images – plus they pay a licencing fee. So, for example, I'll say to a brand 'you can use this for digital purposes, online, for four years, and it'll cost you £100'. Once the four years are up the brand then has to either take the images down or renew the license. But they can also buy the copyright fully, which means they can, for example, sell the images to a stock food website and make revenue off them, alter the images, or use them as part of advertising campaigns. The benefit of the licensing fee is that you can adjust the price according to what the brand is using it for." So, a licencing fee for digital use would usually be considerably lower than for use in a magazine or on a billboard.

Turns out, recipes and copyright are a bit of an interesting (read: complicated) topic; there's actually some debate as to whether a recipe or food creation can be protected by copyright, and what criteria it would need to meet to do so.

In the UK and US, you can't copyright a recipe. The general reason given for this is that a collection of ingredients can't be covered under copyright (in the same way that you can't copyright a list of materials used to build something) and a recipe is a list of instructions, which doesn't fall under the list of things that can be protected by copyright in UK law.

Then we have the case of cookbooks. When these are published, it's with the aim of making them profitable, and you can't easily profit if someone else can just copy and paste the entire book and sell that. This is why, when it comes to cookbooks, copyright law *does* apply. Typographical arrangements are protected, so you can't scan or photocopy the pages without permission or an appropriate licence, which thereby helps to protect the recipes as they are printed. The recipe itself, though, can be copied and pasted, and it's less clear whether this would be a breach of copyright or not. The list of ingredients in a recipe isn't protected, but the wording could be argued to be an 'original literary work'. In practice, this means that while someone could copy the list of ingredients and method, they would need to re-word it to call it their own.

The US Copyright Office official stipulation says: "Mere listings of ingredients as in recipes, formulas, compounds, or prescriptions are not subject to copyright protection. However, when a recipe or formula is accompanied by substantial literary expression in the form of an explanation or directions, or when there is a combination of recipes, as in a cookbook, there may be a basis for copyright protection."

The exception to this rule on recipes is for trade secrets, such as the Coca-Cola recipe or KFC's secret blend of 11 herbs and spices. But, if these recipes were to appear online somewhere, they'd be fair game.

So, a cookbook can be copyrighted, but as a literary work, not a culinary one. It's then considered a work of art.

Images, songs, paintings, stories... these are all protected because they are considered art. Can food be art? Looking on Instagram you could easily think so. The way some people decorate and style their food is certainly a work of art, although from a legal perspective it's only when photographed that it becomes art and is copyrighted. Until you take a picture of your lunch it's not legally art, it's just food. And if you post it online, the social media sites don't own the image that has been posted on their site; the copyright is still retained by you. If a dish has artistic merit separate from its nature as food, the creator may be able to claim they own the rights to it, therefore protecting it from being copied. It seems to be an untested area in UK law, however. I find this particularly fascinating, because it treads the fine line between functional and artistic creations.

Chefs have differing views on this. Dominique Ansel, for example, is quoted as saying, "If anything, food is a more intimate form of art compared to others, as it incorporates all of the senses." Enrique Olvera, on the other hand, says that food isn't so much art, as "more like a craft; not necessarily beautiful, not pretentious, and it doesn't need a statement as long as it nourishes, covers our basic needs, and gives us pleasure. Food's purpose is to see us smile, not to question our existence."

Legal scholar Malla Pollack writes: "Food and art may be related in three different ways. First, an art object may be a representation of a food item. Copyright law has traditionally protected this category as it has protected artistic likenesses of other aspects of the world... Second, food may be used as a medium to create a nonedible physical representation of another object in the real world or the artist's psyche. Consider the chocolate table and chairs (edible materials mounted on plastic frames) exhibited at the American Crafts Museum, or objects created from baker's clay, cornstarch dough, salt dough, or breadcrumb dough... Third, an object may be intended both to be eaten and to appeal to the aesthetic impulse... Members of this category may resemble nonedible objects but most do not look like anything but food. For example, a well-known cookbook is illustrated by reproductions of the chef's own pastel drawings of the food ready to be served. The illustrations are obviously protectable pictorial works."

Overall: the problem with legally protecting recipes lies somewhere between authorship and performance.

The matter of copyright over recipes is complex, and many bloggers have a generally agreed-upon etiquette for navigating this, which Izy described to me. "With a recipe, if you're copying it word for word, maybe consider just linking back to the original post you got it from, because there's really no point you having it on your own website. If you're changing up to 3 things, such as an ingredient, a quantity, or a method, then it's generally considered to be a new recipe. It's not a hard and fast rule, and often it's just good manners to say, 'this recipe is adapted from these sources' even if you change several things."

Of course, it's very easy to develop and write up a recipe that's identical to someone else's by complete coincidence. There are only a limited number of ingredients and combinations in the world, after all. There are also often standard ratios for making foods like a vanilla sponge cake or chocolate chip cookies that you can't deviate too far from before it fails.

Are blogs butchering books?

There are plenty of media articles claiming that blogs are killing the cookbook industry, but statistics show that's not happening at all. The publishing industry has seen a sharp decline in sales, especially when it comes to food magazines, which used to be the easiest way to access recipes, but with the Internet, everything is just a few clicks away. Food magazines have been replaced with blogs that are easily searchable, but cookbooks tell a story, and the recipes collected together mean something.

While I own a kindle, I have never even considered the idea of buying an e-cookbook. Of course, I have no desire to shame those who do, as it can be incredibly convenient, but there's something special and nostalgic about leafing through a cookbook, propping it open in the kitchen and covering it with splatters and stains that are not imperfections but signs of love and use. It's adding your cooking story onto the page and combining it with the author's.

Cookbooks are one of the few areas of the publishing industry that is growing and thriving, and I think blogs and social media are contributing to that. They allow for more diverse voices to be heard, not so much in terms of appearance – almost all fitness and popular food bloggers look pretty much the same, they're often thin, white and middle-class – but in terms of perspectives. Izy agrees, "Before, you were stuck with the regulars – Nigella, Delia, Jamie, and so on – and if you didn't really like their cooking or connect with them, there wasn't really much out there for you. Now, you can find people of different ages, with different styles and aesthetics, so you have far more choice. You can find someone you align with more easily online, and if they bring out a book, you're more likely to buy it."

Of course, the other side of the equation is that bloggers have changed the publishing landscape to a point where some incredibly talented writers and cooks are struggling to get a book deal because they don't have an already established audience.

Fame or talent?

Let's come full circle, back to Julie Powell and Julia Child. Julia's rise in the culinary world is a really inspiring story of hard work and a fight to be recognised for her talent. She was rewarded with fame not because she had insider connections or because she already had a platform where she was well known, but because her work was just that good.

In the movie, *Julie and Julia*, her story is told in tandem with Powell's tale – a tale that we are expected to believe is equivalent and synonymous with Child's. But that's just not the case. In fact, you can argue that the exact opposite is true. Powell wrote a blog documenting her year cooking Child's recipes, and when the *New York Times* ran an article about her, we watch on screen as Powell's answering machine immediately fills up with literary agents and publishers asking her if she's interested in writing a book. When you take a step back from the carefully crafted scene, you realise that these people aren't calling Powell because her blog is so well-written, or because her writing is the Internet equivalent of Child's genuine masterpiece. They're not even calling because she has come up with something innovative. I mean, she's literally replicating someone else's recipes. They are calling because the *New York Times* has said Julie Powell is now famous and has a growing platform of readers who will pay money for her words.

We see this happen over and over again with popular bloggers who can neither cook well nor write well. There are bloggers who have real talent and skill, but they sadly aren't the norm. Some people are rightly concerned that there are more Julia Child-types out there who are genuinely talented and exciting, and who would write fantastic books – books that won't be published because publishers are too busy trying to find the next Julie Powell.

10

HOW IS SOCIAL MEDIA CHANGING THE WORLD?

Internet fame is a strange thing because you can be famous simply for being famous. Amassing fans and followers isn't in itself a notable accomplishment. Getting attention from strangers on the Internet doesn't necessarily mean you've created something of any real value. And yet people can use this fanbase to do good.

When almost every article you read online about social media would have you believe we're all becoming narcissists, it's important to highlight some of the amazing ways people are harnessing social media for good purposes, often being incredibly selfless.

According to a global survey in 2017, 57% of millennial consumers either bought or boycotted brands based on their corporate values. Online activism is rapidly gaining momentum now that we are so connected 24 hours a day, having conversations and sharing ideas. We are using social media to hold our peers accountable and demand better, both from companies and from one another.

Sharing our food stories

Social media has revolutionised our experience of health, in particular. It has fundamentally changed how we find out information about both mental and physical health conditions. What was once highly personal has become extremely public. In some cases, this can be incredibly liberating.

Almost three quarters (72%) of Internet users say they have searched online for health information of one kind or another within the past year, 26% have read about or watched someone else's experience with health or medical issues, and 16% have deliberately tried to find others who experience the same health concerns. This is especially common for those with chronic health conditions – nearly a quarter (23%) have taken their search online to locate others with the same condition.

People search for and share health information online not only for themselves, but also for friends or family members who are struggling. Around half of all online health searches are performed on behalf of someone else. For example, 53% of online health information seekers living with chronic diseases reported that their last online health information search was related to the medical situation of someone else. When we, or someone close to us, are unwell, Dr Google is fast becoming our first port of call.

Special diets

Certain medical conditions require sufferers to exclude foods or eat in a specific way. For example, people with coeliac disease have to avoid all gluten, someone with phenylketonuria (PKU) has to eat a diet low in the amino acid phenylalanine, which also includes avoiding aspartame, the artificial sweetener.

People with special diets use social media for several reasons, including keeping track of illness-related symptoms so they can monitor their responses, finding recipes that are suitable for them, and seeking an online community.

Blogger and content creator Becky Excell struggles with gut health issues that require her to avoid gluten. She uses social media for a variety of reasons. "The biggest thing I share is new recipes. I create recipes that are suitable for those who are gluten-free (but are tasty enough for everyone else too), mainly baking recipes, but also lots of quick and easy meal ideas too. I share gluten-free product finds as well as gluten-free travel guides so that my audience can find places to eat when they are on holiday or a day out." As well as this, she uses her Instagram stories – which disappear after 24 hours – to share more personal information. "I use my Instagram Story to talk more from a real-life perspective about some of my struggles with both mental and physical health. I like to try and keep it as relatable as possible to show others that they are not alone if they also struggle."

The response Becky has had to what she shares online has been overwhelmingly positive. "I get messages on a daily basis from people saying that my gluten-free travel guide was a lifesaver and it made their holiday amazing. I also get so many photographs sent to me of recipes that people have tried out and love. The fact that my audience really seem to relate to me and speak to me as if I was a close friend just makes everything worth it. I really feel like I help a lot of people and that's a special feeling."

What makes social media so suited for talking about special dietary considerations? "I think it's the fact that social media allows you to be able to interact very easily with others. When I want to create a recipe, I can ask my audience for ideas of what they'd like me to create next. When I share a new product find it's instant and within 30 minutes someone who follows me has gone and bought it!"

For Becky, the most important part of sharing all this on social media is the sense of community and understanding. "It's allowed me to meet people who have the same dietary requirements as me, or who have the same gut health issues as me. People that I would never have met outside of social media. I think it's a great place for all of those with special dietary requirements, as many don't have friends or family in a similar position but can feel less alone by finding others all over the world on social media."

And the biggest positive for her? "Definitely the people I've met. I've met some amazing humans who I hope will be friends for life. I would never have met them without my blog and social media. Social media and the positive feedback I get when people like what I post has given me so much confidence in myself (which is something I truly lack). The opportunities outside of social media have been amazing too: I've travelled abroad, been on live national radio numerous times, spoken at events and done live cooking demos, to name a few. None of this would have been possible without social media."

Mental health conversations

Social media may be contributing to a number of mental health issues such as depression, anxiety and eating disorders, but it is also being used as a tool to raise awareness. In the midst of all the 'perfect life' accounts online, some people are deliberately defying that and making themselves vulnerable by sharing their everyday mental health struggles. Many people choose to hide this part of themselves, and I have no intention of judging them for doing so. I understand why people wouldn't want to share; mental health is a very personal thing, and sharing should be a personal choice. Especially when faced with the social comparison and shaming of social media platforms, why would you want to put yourself through that?

One of the most well-known examples of someone who defies this is the novelist and journalist Matt Haig, author of many bestselling books including *Reasons to Stay Alive* (2015). This book, and the way he talks so candidly about his emotions and experiences, have helped countless people feel seen, and likely even helped people find their own reasons to stay alive rather than consider suicide. Social media is instant, and because we've made a habit of accessing it often when we feel at our worst, I can think of no better place for individuals like Matt to write and share.

Chartered psychologist Kimberley Wilson says one of the best things she's seen online is the destigmatisation of therapy. "I have been thrilled to see the number of fitness influencers who are talking positively about their experiences with therapy! Though therapy is necessarily private it shouldn't be taboo, and I think it is great that these individuals are using their platforms to demystify and destigmatise psychological therapy."

More people than we realise live with mental health conditions, and on social media increasing numbers of those who do share their stories help to make others feel less alone, which is a truly wonderful thing.

Positive messages about food and exercise

Speaking of fitness bloggers, one of the great shifts that has been happening online recently is personal trainers shifting their message from purely fat loss to a broader picture of health and exercise, that isn't purely focused on aesthetics.

There are huge benefits to exercising that have nothing to do with weight. In addition, we have research looking at #fitspo images and body image that shows that these images, which focus heavily on someone's shape, are making people feel worse about themselves, and don't actually encourage people to exercise more. Thankfully, this shift in message has been slowly making its way to the masses on social media over the last few years. Tally Rye is one of those people leading the charge.

"I make the content I wish was there and I had seen a few years ago. Most of my content comes from conversations I have with people, whether online or offline. I want people to feel like they are being educated on the benefits of exercise that aren't centred around aesthetics or weight loss. I want people to move more, and to encourage people to exercise, and to do so for the right reasons."

Why does she want people to move away from aesthetics? "Through my own personal experience, I found that focusing on aesthetics didn't work for me long term, and actually led me to have the worst body image I'd ever had. The more I focused on something the more I picked myself apart, and when I was at my leanest and most #fitspo I was at my most preoccupied with food, my body, fitness, but I didn't really have a life, and was really insecure about how I looked. I was peak #fitspo but

I was so unhappy. The less #fitspo I look now, the happier I am, because I'm not so preoccupied with my body."

Some people build their brand around their body. There are fitness bloggers who build their entire brand around their bum. And fair play to them for being successful with that! But it's also great to see some fitness professionals using social media to move away from this heavy focus on appearance.

Tally agrees, "I hear so many fitness bloggers saying 'I have to post bikini pictures to talk about the important stuff otherwise no one is going to read it. I have to clickbait'. No, you don't. I stopped clickbaiting and I started doing what felt right for me so I could sleep at night, and my follower count went up, I got a book deal, and great things have happened in my career."

People being more comfortable and accepting of their bodies can only be a good thing. People who accept and appreciate their bodies, no matter their shape or size, are more likely to treat their bodies with respect, which means they're more likely to engage in healthy behaviours like eating a varied nutritious diet, moving their bodies, and getting enough sleep. They're also more likely to have better overall mental health, and it's important we remember that good mental health is just as important as good physical health.

Countering misinformation online

The Internet and social media are where quacks and charlatans thrive. Qualifications don't matter anywhere near as much online as having a pretty face and giving people simple narratives to follow. People like the Medical Medium, who don't have a single shred of expertise or evidence, gain millions of followers by sharing soundbites like 'parsley removes aluminium from the body' and 'asparagus dislodges fat cells from the liver'. Social media is where misinformation thrives.

The fact that anyone could create an account and say anything was once hailed as the most exciting thing about social media, and yet such democratisation can be exactly what causes the problem. Anyone can create an account, claim they're an expert, and start giving out advice. Even when there is no malicious intent, even when people just want to help, that doesn't mean they're not to blame for any adverse outcomes. Nutrition is one of those areas where everyone thinks they're an expert because they eat every day and they're still alive. Eating food doesn't make you qualified to tell others what to eat, in the same way that playing Grand Theft Auto doesn't qualify you to be a driving instructor.

And yet, there is hope! There are growing numbers of health-care professionals and academics turning to social media to counter the woo. I mean, I've accidently built a career on it. In the United States, one hospital is taking the fight against online misinformation very seriously. Dr Austin Chiang is a gastroenterologist who studied at Harvard, and now holds the position of Chief Medical Social Media Officer at the Thomas Jefferson University Hospital in Philadelphia. It is the first position of its kind. Part of his job is to get doctors and other health professionals on social media to drown out health misinformation by posting their own content that is fact-checked, accurate and helpful for patients. Every few days Dr Chiang posts a picture of himself and his work with details about the latest research or advice to patients trying to navigate health information online.

Dr Joshua Wolrich is another example of a doctor who has a talent for countering health misinformation online, which has gained him a large following. I asked him what his motivation is:

"Social media is perfect for sharing information in bite-size chunks, but this can also add to the problem of misinformation. References and evidence are rarely as expected as they would be in a news article or peer-reviewed journal, and this makes it very easy for people to share opinion as fact. Combining that with the virality of social media creates the perfect medium for concern."

I definitely agree with this, and neither myself nor Dr Wolrich are inclined to stay quiet. "Misinformation isn't addressed through silence, it can't be. I also believe it very important to notice the medium through which it is being spread. When it occasionally feels like I'm fighting a losing battle, it's the regular messages from followers that remind me why I can't stop. The overwhelming positive response each time I address even the most obvious nonsense is an encouragement that it's a privilege to be able to sift through the misinformation without underlying anxiety. When a member of the public comes across an anti-vaccine post online, they are rarely going to have the time or expertise to do a literature search and work out which opposing view is true. Instead, credible professionals need to start joining and using social media to correct misinformation. Do we really expect things to change by turning a blind eye? It won't. It's time to start putting that authority bias to good."

It seems we agree: social media is an incredibly vital tool for the countering of misinformation. And many healthcare professionals are now joining in as well, from Dr Anjali Mahto (who you met in chapter 4), a consultant dermatologist who counters misinformation on subjects like acne and skincare, to Dr Jen

Gunter who is leading the battle against Goop and their crazy obsession with telling people to stick things up their vaginas. All of these people do incredible work, and I recommend you follow them all.

I don't for a second believe that shouting down the opposition online is enough, but healthcare professionals and scientists have to meet the charlatans where they're at, and use the same platforms they do. In the world of food and nutrition, there is no knowledge deficit – people are overloaded with information and confused about what to eat. But I have to believe that if enough of us share the evidence, consistently, then it can make a difference. Otherwise, what's the point?

I receive messages each week from people who tell me that my social media posts have helped them unfollow quacks, ignore sensationalist headlines, and focus on what the experts are saying. While it can sometimes feel disheartening to speak up in the face of so much pseudoscience, they are a nice reminder that it's all worth it.

I do believe that the responsibility regarding misinformation online goes three ways. It belongs to the consumers, the professionals, and to the platforms themselves. Thankfully, these platforms are starting to step up to the demand from both politicians, public health, and from consumers of social media.

In 2018 Pinterest realised that the search results for many health-related terms were being overwhelmed with misinformation. When people searched for 'vaccines' the anti-vaxxer rhetoric appeared, and searches for 'cancer cure' came up with all sorts of unproven and illegal remedies. In response to this, they decided to take a drastic step and broke the search function for those terms. If someone searched those words, a message would appear on an otherwise blank screen saying, "If you're looking for medical advice, please contact a healthcare provider".

In 2019, Pinterest took this another step further, to redouble their efforts at fighting misinformation. Users are now able to search for terms related to vaccines, but the results displayed will only come from major public health organisations, including the World Health Organization (WHO), Centre for Disease Control, American Academy of Paediatrics (AAP) and Vaccine Safety Net.

Most of the major social media platforms have adopted new policies toward anti-vaccine misinformation in response to pressure from public health organisations, politicians and the media. Facebook, for example, has begun to reduce the reach of groups and pages that spread anti-vaccination rhetoric, including removing some of them entirely. YouTube has moved anti-vaccine videos into a category of 'harmful' misinformation videos that are not promoted by its recommendation algorithm, which limits their reach.

All social media platforms have taken time to combat pro-anorexia content to protect their users. Instagram, Facebook, Pinterest and Tumblr, which are all extremely visual outlets, have made very public vows to create online spaces free from pro-ED (eating disorder) content. So far, they're doing OK. Instagram has apparently displayed health warnings for search terms encouraging eating disorders since 2012. If you search #bulimia or #anorexia, for instance, the app will offer to connect you to resources that can help. Searches for #proana, #thinspiration, or #bonespo (used for 'inspiring' images of people with visible bones) won't show any results at all, even though the tags are still widely in use.

I hope in the future that these platforms will start to take more action when it comes to other areas of health misinformation as well, such as food and nutrition. One small step has already recently occurred – thanks to social media campaigning by actress Jameela Jamil and others, Instagram no longer allows detox tea images to be shown to under 18s. Yes, she was also in talks with Instagram behind the scenes, but the support she received online was a huge contributing factor. It just goes to show that social media platforms are capable of making these decisions, even if it pisses off a small percentage of their consumers, for the protection of the overall group. They just need to get it done.

When scientific journals are complicit

Alan Flanagan, a PhD student in nutrition, says the following: "Social media has become a tool for perpetuating misleading information, even extending to the conduct of academic journals. The *British Journal of Sports Medicine* serves as an unsavoury example of where academic integrity succumbs to an agenda. Although there is an ethical duty to report research results fairly and transparently, the *BJSM* became a vehicle to promote an anti-guideline, pro-high-fat, cholesterol-denialist narrative in the public discourse. One article, provocatively entitled 'Saturated fat does not clog the arteries: coronary heart disease is a chronic inflammatory condition, the risk of which can be effectively reduced from healthy lifestyle interventions', became the most retweeted post of the *BJSM* social media pages, and most read editorial."

So, what role did social media play in all this? "The lead author of the article, a UK-based cardiologist named Aseem Malhotra, leveraged the *BJSM* and social media to perpetuate an anti-statin rhetoric which was associated with an 11 and 12% increase in the likelihood of members of the public discontinuing statin therapy for primary and secondary prevention, respectively. This level of discontinued treatment would be predicted to result in over 2,000 more cardiovascular events in the UK over a 10-year period. Indeed, it was via Twitter that a number of academics petitioned the journal to publish a rebuttal, after its repeated refusal to do so. Thus, social media has become an arena where the traditional issues of research misconduct – data falsification, fabrication, misreporting methodology, misrepresentation of results and plagiarism – have been expanded into the ability to use opinion framed as research to have profound negative impacts on population health. The *BJSM/BMJ* and Malhotra serve as examples of how this can happen."

Scientific process isn't infallible, because it is humans who do science and who publish research, and humans are inherently flawed. When misinformation occurs, scientific journals have a duty to correct this, not simply ignore it because it was popular on social media. Online reach should never be seen as more important than scientific accuracy. Thankfully, academics on social media can use the very same platforms to demand change.

For the health of the planet

It would be wrong to spend an entire book talking about food and social media without discussing how people online are trying to change our eating habits for the health of the planet.

Climate change is a fact, one I have no desire to debate, and which must be recognised for its significance on our future.

While it can sometimes feel like not much is being done on a larger scale, there are individuals and groups with an audience who are using their social media platforms to try and do something good.

Carmen Huter is a travel photographer who shares important messages about the environment on her social media in the captions for her unbelievably stunning images. She says, "My world travels and personal health problems allowed me to educate myself on all things sustainability. For instance, I saw first-hand what climate change does to wild animals in the Kenyan savannah. I learnt how ethnic minorities in Vietnam have a very cyclical and holistic relationship with where their food comes from; being part of every step of the process. I also realised the great opportunity that lies within motivating those around us to action and aspiring to positive change as a group rather than an individual."

Carmen credits social media for shaping her understanding of what it means to have a balanced diet that also considers planetary health. "Social media has led me to be inspired by a multitude of creatives and entrepreneurs around this world. Some of them work in the food space, pushing boundaries on what it means to have a 'normal' well-balanced diet. They transformed the language of the typical meat and three veg standard, or, rather, broadened its terms to include plant-based and wholesome options. In this way, it has introduced me to new ways of putting meals together."

What I love most about Carmen, though, and why I specifically wanted to speak to her, is that she isn't vegan, but describes her diet as 'vegan-ish'. She explains, "I am not fully vegan because I have come to learn that my body thrives off a variety of foods, especially those that are high in healthy fats and proteins. To allow me to feel both comfortable and well-nourished while I travel to dozens of different countries every year, I find that I instead prioritise eating local, fresh and wholesome food as opposed to vegan only. This means I consume local fish and, once in a blue moon, dairy. Ultimately, I feel more fuelled, less pressured to try and find food I am safe to eat and more comfortable in my travels." Just to be clear, I applaud anyone who is able to and decides to go vegan for the planet, but I also think it's wonderful that there are environmental activists and role models who are more flexible with this approach and are comfortable sharing this, as the backlash online can be significant. Carmen has experienced some of this herself. She says she receives pushback "every now and then", but not often. She shares, "It's easy for people to think in black and white and give me a hard time for eating NZ salmon or god knows whatever lands on my story. But that's OK, and I don't take it to heart unless it has depth and value."

Carmen sees the work she does online as activism. Through her words and images she has inspired other people to take a closer look at what they eat: "From the feedback I receive, I can tell many people have opened themselves up to education around where our food comes from and how it's made. I hope to also encourage my audience to understand the impact that what we eat has on the planet. It's a privilege to inspire a more educated and wholesome take on food."

Social media is an ideal platform for this kind of work. "Social media offers the ability to directly communicate to a vast number of people who are engaged, keen to create positive change and, most importantly, curious," says Carmen. I totally agree – the curiosity people have online is, I believe, greater than in the real world, because of the anonymity afforded by social media. People can explore ideas and opinions without the pressure of someone watching and judging.

At the beginning of May 2019, a UN panel on biodiversity published a report on food waste. In the report, they named food waste as a major contributor towards rising carbon emissions.

It is estimated that one-third of all edible food produced for global human consumption is lost or wasted each year – a truly shocking statistic. Around 10 million tonnes of food and drink were wasted in the food chain in 2015, which is equivalent to around one-quarter of the 41 million tonnes of food bought that year. Around 60% of this is avoidable, meaning that it was edible but simply no longer wanted or past its best-before date. This doesn't include things like eggshells or banana skins, which aren't really edible. In 2015 the average UK household with children spent £60 per month on food that could have been eaten but instead was thrown away. This has economic impacts, as food waste exacerbates rising food prices globally, causing food to be less attainable to the poorest people in the world. This has a direct social impact by increasing the number of mal-nourished people.

Arguably the most damaging impact of vast levels of food waste is the environmental effect. Production of food that is consequently wasted adds pressure onto the diminishing for-ests that are inevitably altered for agricultural land – if this food wasn't wasted, then perhaps less land would be needed to feed the same number of people. Additionally, the disposal of food waste to landfill adds to the avoidable release of gases like methane and carbon dioxide.

Companies face a challenging task of trying to ask their customers to consume less, or at least to consume differently, which is difficult for companies with a high-volume economic business model. Companies rely on profit, which generally requires increasing the quantity of sales, not trying to reduce it. There are, however, incentives for companies to focus on the environmental impacts, as it can inspire stronger customer brand loyalty. Especially in younger generations, there is an increasing awareness of climate change, and a company who is seen to consider this as an important component of their business model is more likely to be seen favourably. The environmentally aware are no longer are no longer a niche group, but a considerable percentage of the population.

One such experiment was conducted with the supermarket ASDA in the UK. Information about reducing food waste was offered in the supermarket's magazine and in their email newsletter, while on their Facebook page customers were asked to share their favourite recipes that used leftover food. All three locations also directed people to other resources on reducing food waste. In the end, all three tactics resulted in consumers wasting less food, but the Facebook page had the additional benefit of being interactive and getting consumers involved, rather than just talking at them.

While household food waste is a significantly larger proportion of overall food waste than that of companies – retailers produce less than 3% of food waste in the UK – that doesn't absolve them of any and all responsibility.

A number of social media campaigns have attempted to

highlight how much food is wasted by large companies, in particular how much food is refused by supermarkets for being 'ugly'. Hashtags such as #UglyIsBeautiful and #LoveTheUgly are trying to encourage consumers to buy food that doesn't look perfect and encourage supermarkets to sell this food. After all, the shape of a tomato doesn't really impact its flavour, and once you chop carrots into cubes it doesn't matter how straight they were. If you're making soup or a smoothie or anything else that involves blending produce, why should you care what shape it is? When we grow food ourselves we enjoy and laugh at the weird and wonderful shapes fruits and vegetables can make – we celebrate them. We shouldn't treat supermarket produce any different.

As a result of the pressure from consumers, particularly online, a number of UK supermarkets now offer 'wonky' products in many large stores at cheaper prices than the prettier versions. Asda sells 'wonky veg boxes', Tesco sells 'wonky' produce, Morrisons does a 'wonky vegetables selection box', Lidl offer 'too good to waste' boxes of slightly damaged and bruised produce, and Waitrose have their 'a little less than perfect' collection of produce.

So far, all this awareness around food waste seems to be working. At the household level, people now waste 1 million tonnes of food per year less than they did in 2007. But we can't just focus on one aspect.

At the other end of the process, activists are using social media to showcase the treasures they uncover from dumpster diving, or to use their preferred name, freeganism*. Many are not

---

* 'Freegan' is an amalgamation of the words 'free' and 'vegan', as they don't pay for the items, and it has similar concepts to veganism by trying to be kinder to the planet. Freeganism encompasses dumpster diving, trading, foraging, gardening and sharing.

doing this for financial reasons but to fight the system of over-consumption. Some have large freezers where they store all this food, some make food that they donate to soup kitchens, and others distribute it around their neighbourhood.

By sharing their finds on social media, they aim to educate the public on how much perfectly edible food is thrown away, so it's no longer 'out of sight, out of mind'. The large flatlays of all the food can be quite impressive, especially when the pictures show extreme hauls such as over 80 corn on the cob, 40 bags of Lindt chocolate, or 35 plastic bottles of ketchup, all from a single supermarket. We are visual creatures after all, and seeing that many ketchup bottles is a lot more shocking than imagining them.

One woman goes through the trash of a US pharmacy in New York a few times a week. She started a petition to ask them to change their policy to donate more of their products, including food, rather than throw them away. Over 300,000 people have signed the petition. Apparently, many retailers are afraid of donating food because they don't want to be sued if the food is slightly off, but the Good Samaritan Food Donation Act, signed in 1996, protects food donors from liability in the case of harm or illness. So far, there have been no recorded lawsuits related to food donation.

In 2019, more than 100 of the biggest players in the food industry, including all of the UK's major supermarkets, signed a government pledge to halve their food waste by 2030. I hope they succeed.

This is an example of how individual and group action on social media can lead to real change, and potentially even reach government and impact policy. More on that in the next chapter.

11

HOW IS SOCIAL MEDIA CHANGING FOOD POLICY?

Politics and policy don't often come up in conversations centred around nutrition. There is a huge focus on individual responsibility, as evidenced by the vast number of diet books that give you a list of foods to eat and a list of foods to avoid. We like the idea that we are in charge of our own decisions and that we have control.

We do have some control, yes, but there are many other factors that shape our food decisions, including our food environment. Our individual needs and preferences have to compete with the desires of the food industry, and the two don't always match up. At that point, an individual can easily feel powerless when trying to stand up to large corporations, and in those cases putting pressure on the industry via government policy can be an effective solution.

Social media has played a considerable role in shaping the conversation around public health and nutrition policy.

Importantly, it's a way to engage the public and create an appetite for change.

With the examples I'm going to give, my goal isn't to come down on one side or another, to say whether these campaigns are good or bad. My intention is simply to offer them up as examples of how powerful a tool social media can be when used to create change.

The 'sugar tax'

In 2015, celebrity chef and campaigner Jamie Oliver released a documentary called *Sugar Rush*, in which he looked at the effects sugar has on the health of the population. What he discovered angered and saddened him to the point that he created a petition to introduce a tax on sugary drinks. That petition spread on social media and had 155,516 signatures – easily exceeding the 100,000 mark needed for the issue to be considered for parliamentary debate.

That September, parliament responded to the petition, saying: "The Government has no plans to introduce a tax on sugar-sweetened beverages. The Government has committed to a tax lock to avoid raising the cost of living and to promote UK productivity and economic growth, however, the Government keeps all taxes under review, with decisions being a matter for the Chancellor as part of the Budget process. The causes of obesity are complex, caused by a number of dietary, lifestyle, environmental and genetic factors, and tackling it will require a comprehensive and broad approach. As such, the Government is considering a range of options for tackling childhood obesity, and the contribution that Government, alongside industry, families and communities can make, and will announce its plans for tackling childhood obesity by the end of the year."

Parliament debated the topic in November 2015, and in 2016 it was announced that the government would be introducing a Soft Drinks Industry Levy – more commonly known as the 'sugar tax' – in 2018. The two-year period was to give the industry time for reformulation, so they could change their recipes to have less sugar, and thereby avoid or reduce the amount of tax paid, which wasn't insignificant: 24 pence per litre if it contains 8 grams of sugar per 100 millilitres, and 18 pence per litre if it contains 5–8 grams of sugar per 100 millilitres. This tax is paid by the manufacturers directly, with on average around a third being passed on to the consumer.

Naturally, there has been some backlash to this, amid concerns about the cost being passed on to consumers and thereby affecting the poorest populations the most. There has also been considerable anger from consumers who disliked the taste of the reformulated products, and who didn't want to have the choice of sugar or artificial sweeteners taken away from them. A new petition entitled 'Hands off our IRN BRU' received almost 55,000 signatures, mostly from angry Scots.*

There's no denying that social media had a significant impact on the tax coming into fruition. The tax was backed by 69% of the public, which showed the government that this was something that the majority wanted, and would therefore be in their best interests if they wanted to remain in power.

---

* Irn-Bru is basically Scotland's national drink, second to whisky of course. In Scotland, Irn-Bru even outsells Coca-Cola.

If you're wondering whether a policy change was really needed for this, as it turns out, probably yes. Jenny Rosborough, a registered public health nutritionist, says: "When it comes to food and nutrition-related policies to change the food environment, it has become clear that we need the government to step in and legislate to create a level playing field amongst food and drinks manufacturers to ensure change occurs across the board and impacts hard-to-reach populations who are likely to benefit the most. And conversations on social media can help reassure the government that there is public appetite for intervention. The Soft Drinks Industry Levy, which is essentially a mandatory sugar reduction programme whereby manufacturers are taxed on products containing more than 5% sugar, is a great example of this. Sugar reduction in the first two years has been ten times greater than that of the government's voluntary sugar reduction programme in food. However, in the absence of legislation, the media is a key vehicle used to catalyse change and hold industry to account."

Data analysed in 2020 shows that there has been a 29% reduction of sugar per 100 millilitres in soft drinks. The soft drinks market is as large as ever, but it seems, so far, the tax may be working.

#AdEnough

In 2018, Jamie Oliver came out with a new campaign, with the aim of protecting children from junk food marketing. He proposed a 9 p.m. watershed for these kinds of adverts on television: "Currently, there's nothing in place to protect our kids from seeing these adverts – apart from literally covering their eyes! And that's where our #AdEnough campaign comes in..."

He came up with a simple hashtag: #AdEnough, which he asked people to share on social media alongside a picture of themselves hiding their eyes. Simple, clear, easy to do. At the time of writing, the government had opened a consultation to get the views of the public from March to June 2019, and we are waiting to hear their response. Online polling apparently shows that 70% of respondents support a 9 p.m. watershed on junk food adverts online, so it could go the same way as the sugar tax.

In the meantime, a related change occurred: Transport for London banned junk food advertisements on the London Underground, Overground, buses, Docklands Light Railway, taxis and bus stops. Essentially, every form of public transport in London. The ban is aimed at high fat, salt and sugar (HFSS) food and drinks, which are defined by Public Health England's guidelines. On the day it was enforced, an image circulated on social media saying "Sadiq Khan [The Mayor of London] has #AdEnough of junk food ads on Transport for London."

Jenny Rosborough wrote this on her Instagram regarding the campaign: "From today, only adverts for food and drinks that are not high in fat, sugar, salt (HFSS) will be allowed to be advertised across Transport for London. Research has shown, in children, that HFSS food and drink marketing is associated with increased preference, immediate snack food consumption, greater intake of HFSS products, increased food intake that is not compensated for at later meals, and weight gain. This sets a great precedent – for other cities but also for a future where it's not the norm to see unhealthy food adverts on every corner."

It's still relatively early days, but data suggests that this ban had led to a change in the advertisements being shown without loss of revenue for Transport for London.

There's now another hashtag floating around: #NotForChildren with calls to ban the sales of energy drinks to under 16-year-olds. These energy drinks often specify 'not for children' on the packaging, which inspired the hashtag and made it easier to remember.

We also have the newly created #BiteBack2030, a campaign asking influencers to stop promoting junk food due to the concerns about how children respond to influencer marketing, and in the hope that this can encourage them towards more nutrient-dense food choices. The website includes an open letter to influencers, which people are encouraged to sign. The letter reads: 'Dear Influencers, Everyday [sic] we see your pictures, we like, we comment, we share; we support you. Now we are asking you to support us. Underneath the filters and fine-tuning of your posts, you are just like me, a normal person. That's precisely why people follow, trust and listen to what you have to say, and why over half of us teens have bought something endorsed by a YouTuber. It's also why, if we see vloggers promoting sugary snacks, studies show we will eat 25% more of that food (that isn't good for us) than we would've otherwise. As your name suggests, you are in a powerful position and now we need you.' The letter then goes on to ask influencers to use their online presence to promote healthier options.

This is the first time a public health campaign has focused so specifically on influencers and highlights how much of a role they can play in determining food choice. Guess who's behind it? Jamie Oliver, of course.

How does it work?

Social media can contribute to changing policy through a combination of three tactics:

Putting on the pressure

From talking to various public health and policy experts, I've come to realise that in order to get traction in parliament you need media traction. While healthcare professionals will have their nuanced perspectives, marketing teams understandably want to generate noise through dramatic headlines that capture the public's attention. Without this, it's incredibly difficult to bring things to the attention of parliament. While the media is important for articulating these messages, what amplifies this further and spreads it faster is the public response on social media.

The recent focus on sugar was the vehicle for changing food policy and forcing the food industry to join in. In 2015, the UK government guidelines changed to recommend that only 5% of our daily energy intake comes from added sugar. Guidelines rarely change, because it takes significant evidence to warrant that (as it should), so this was a huge deal that opened up the conversation around sugar and health. Sugar was at the forefront of people's minds, and enabled a discussion around how the food industry can change to help people meet this new target for added sugar intake.

The point of the sugar-reduction programme, which focuses on reformulation of recipes, was to put the onus on manufacturers and the food industry to reduce the amount of sugar in their products where they are able to. But in order to keep the pressure on the government and food manufacturers you have to gain media traction – no one likes bad press – and social media facilitates the spread of these articles.

A large conversation on social media, from both individuals and from groups, provides great leverage. This is best done through a specific campaign and a message, for example the hashtag #AdEnough. When these hashtags start trending they appear in the sidebar of people's newsfeeds, attracting even more attention.

Well thought-out strategies and campaigns, with a hashtag and very specific messages, can garner a lot of support and can put real pressure on legislators.

Accessible politicians

Our elected officials are more accessible to us than ever before. You can now directly tweet your MP or congressman, something that would have been unthinkable even twenty years ago. People have full conversations (and sometimes arguments) with politicians on social media and voice their concerns to them directly. Many politicians even have blogs where you can find out exactly what they're thinking and you can share your thoughts.

Jenny Rosborough adds: "[Social media] gives us direct access to MPs, the policymakers, the food and drink industry and millions of members of the general public. Responsible celebrities with a social purpose – who are being informed by qualified nutrition professionals – can also be a force for good in amplifying key messages."

True, a celebrity retweet can sometimes be the key difference to help a message spread quickly across the Internet.

Social media is enhancing the transfer of evidence from academia to policymakers and allows politicians to find out what their constituents think in real-time. Backed up and cross referenced by other data sources, it presents a powerful opportunity for public policymakers and service providers to develop a rich source of real-time, reliable data about social, economic and political issues.

Data and more data

If you ask a food company to change their products and potentially lose profit, they're very unlikely to do it. Understandably so, they're a business and money matters. But if you can create a case for consumer demand, and/or collect polling data to present to government about what people want to see, then they start to pay attention.

You can shout on social media, you can tweet at politicians, but in the end, they want to be re-elected. They want to know that publicly supporting or opposing something will get voters on their side. For that, you need proof. You need numbers and data.

Polling data is one option, another is to present a petition. "The Soft Drinks Industry Levy made the government agenda as a result of a petition – shared and amplified via social media," says Jenny Rosborough. "Within minutes it had reached the 10,000 signatures required to trigger a response from Government; and within a little over 48 hours it had surpassed 100,000 signatures needed to be considered for debate in Parliament." Those are significant numbers, enough to make any politician pay attention.

Social media has changed petitions forever. Gone are the days when you had to create a hugely expensive TV advert or have people wandering the streets with a pen and paper; you just have to retweet and sign. You can reach huge numbers of people so much more easily and cheaply. Many of us feel uncomfortable about having someone with a clipboard or representing a charity approach us in the street, and actively try to avoid them by keeping our head down, wearing headphones, or taking a detour. (I do this too, it's OK to admit it.) We resent this intrusion into our time and space. But on social media we have no issues with tweets and posts appearing asking us to get involved with something, as we feel it's voluntary, private, and something we can think about at our leisure. We feel like we're doing a good thing because we want to, not because someone in the street has put us on the spot with witnesses.

Since the official UK Parliament petitions website was set up in 2015, e-petitions have become an ingrained feature of the British political system, not to mention most people's social media feeds. The system offers the general public a direct route to raise their concerns and outrages with those in power. Any British citizen can start a petition, which is reviewed by the Petitions Committee. They select petitions of interest to find out more about the issues raised and have the power to press for action from government or Parliament.

Petitions are one clear way of demonstrating consumer demand, and hashtags are another. While there may be many people all talking about the same thing online, you can't easily track it as they are all using their own words and phrasing. A hashtag, on the other hand, allows you to collect useful data on exactly how many people have used it, giving a good indication of how many people care about a particular topic. Twitter, like other social media platforms, has an analytics system where they track and follow hashtags. Through this, they can share the top ten hashtags with every user in the world, in your country, or in the chosen area of the follower, as well. On the home page, Twitter displays the 'trends' and 'moments' for all to see and click on. A hashtag takes all these individual posts, tweets and conversations and turns them into a tangible number that can be used to prove the people are interested in the subject and care.

If the data comes from polls, or you have statistics from social media about what consumers think, you have numbers you can present, and the large numbers of engagement on social media can be impressive. Food companies or politicians may worry about backlash against something like the sugar tax (which they definitely did worry about), but being presented with clear numbers that they can work with reassures them the public is on their side.

And the numbers do add up. "Often policies are seen to happen *to* people, not with them. But social media allows the public to be part of the conversation and consumer voice is a key asset," says Jenny Rosborough. "For example, Twitter traction led to enough signatures on a petition to have the Soft Drinks Industry Levy (the 'sugar tax') debated in Parliament. This message also filtered through to the soft drinks industry. The public wanted less sugar in their drinks and consumer demand, aside from regulation, is one of the best ways to trigger change."

Social media provides users with a low-cost yet highly effective method to rally support around causes that they believe to be important, and it offers a way for individuals to put forward new ideas to a large and often receptive audience.

Hashtag activism

Cynics argue that we are living through an age of 'hashtag activism' – a term coined by the media, which refers to the use of hashtags for Internet activism. Critics argue that because it's so easy to retweet, like or share something, that leads to people thinking they've done something useful when in reality they haven't helped. They argue that people are publicly indicating they care about something rather than actually doing something that leads to real change.

It's true that simply starting a petition isn't a guarantee that change will happen – some of the largest petitions created, with millions of signatures, have been rejected by government after all – but where it can really make a difference is when a petition is based around issues that might not otherwise have won much media or parliamentary attention, but which matter a great deal to a large number of people.

What about in the United States? Around half of Americans engage in some form of political or social-minded activity on social media during the year. The majority of Americans think social media is important for getting elected officials to pay attention to issues or for initiating sustained social movements. US researchers examined state residents' past social media posts and these scholars found they could predict whether a proposed policy measure would pass 'with approximately 80% accuracy'. This accuracy is actually greater than predictions made through the use of polling data. It lends itself to the theory that, yes, social media really does have a substantial effect on the law, and that we should be paying attention to it.

People who simply 'like' content while sitting on their sofa binge-watching *Game of Thrones* aren't activists, they're simply social media enthusiasts who spend a lot of time online and show their support for things they agree with.

People who are activists offline tend to use social media activism as a way to build support and organise others into taking the fight offline and into the real world. They are the ones committed to a cause, who become part of a movement and stick to the issue until there is change, not just signing off once they've added their name to a petition. These are activists who know the power of social media and use it as a tool to further their cause. They are the real social media activists.

Hopefully I've shown you that online social media activism can produce change. Petitions can lead to parliamentary debates on issues they might not otherwise have taken seriously. Policy campaigners and public health professionals can use social media statistics, including those from hashtags and online polls, to convince the government to create new laws and take action.

Harnessing social media for behaviour change

Considering the power social media can have, and all this knowledge about how social media affects our food choices, it's unsurprising that researchers have tried to take advantage of this by using social media to reach and engage with young people. In particular, to try and reach those who may not otherwise seek out healthcare professionals in more traditional settings. Young people are more likely to Google something and search for advice online than immediately book a doctor's appointment.

According to a survey by the Pew Research Center, 42% of American adult social media users state that information they find via social media would affect health decisions related to diet, exercise or stress management. Nearly 90% of people aged 18–24 years have indicated they would trust medical information found on social media. That's a lot of people.

Despite all this, it seems that using social media for the site of health interventions doesn't seem to effectively change behaviour. "Social media can be a really useful tool for creating awareness around food research findings, nutrition guidelines and recipe sharing," observes Jenny Rosborough, "however, for many people, behaviour change depends on more than receiving information; our eating patterns are influenced by several factors. Many public health nutrition policies are designed to nudge and enable consumers into engaging in healthier behaviours which is an indirect, but valuable, use of social media."

This doesn't stop researchers and organisations from trying, though. It seems social media is only effective in this way when individuals actively make the decision to follow someone or search for something, not when that content is forced upon us. We want to feel that we are making a choice for ourselves. What this means is that (surprise, surprise) it matters who you choose to follow. It matters what information you seek out on social media. It also means you have some power there, which you can use to your own advantage.

The Royal Society for Public Health (RSPH) has a campaign called Scroll Free September. The idea is that people delete their social media apps for 30 days in order to reassess how they feel, and see if they want to change their relationship with social media as a result. An All-Party Parliamentary Group (APP.) on Social

Media and Young People's Mental Health and Wellbeing has been established by the RSPH to 'drive policy change that mitigates the negatives and maximises the positives of social media for young people'. The APP. is, understandably, concerned by the amount of time young people spend on social media, and how this can impact their health. The group aims to build on the current available evidence suggesting social media can have a significant impact on young people's mental health and wellbeing. They also intend to increase awareness of the issue among politicians, and to drive policy change to mitigate some of the negatives of social media, while encouraging the positives. The group has recently launched an inquiry into how to manage the impact of social media on young people's mental health and wellbeing. So, who knows, soon we might have official policy on social media use.

There's always a downside

"Social media gives everyone a platform. When it comes to public health you have a range of voices; from academics, health professionals and policymakers to the food and drink industry, consumer rights forums and the general public. It can be really helpful to listen to other perspectives," explains Jenny Rosborough. "But there is also the issue of misinformation from authoritative voices. Policymaking is tactical and there have been examples in public health whereby social media has been used to spread inaccurate messages to the detriment of health policies."

One such example of where inaccurate messages have been spread on social media is in the recent 'debates' on saturated fat.

I put that word in quotations because there has been no change in the body of evidence around the effects of saturated fat on our health, and this has been confirmed in a 2019 report by the Scientific Advisory Committee on Nutrition (SACN), which reviewed the evidence on the relationship between saturated fats, health outcomes and risk factors for chronic conditions such as type-2 diabetes and heart disease in the UK population. The report states: 'It is recommended that the dietary reference value for saturated fats remains unchanged.' In other words, the report reaffirmed the UK government's guidelines to limit the overall saturated fat in our diets.

On social media, however, the story is a little different. Remember the cardiologist and cholesterol denier Aseem Malhotra? We're back to him again. He has pushed the narrative that saturated fat is harmless and that carbohydrates are the real issue (that's not how it works), and his Twitter rants have given him a frightening amount of power. Not content with talking in medical schools around the country about how statins are killing everyone, he has befriended a few members of parliament. Most notably, Tom Watson, former Deputy Leader of the Labour Party.* Watson claims he lost considerable amounts of weight and reversed his type-2 diabetes by following the advice from Aseem's book, which pushes the low-carb diet and claims that the reason people in Pioppi in southern Italy live so long is because they eat low-carb. Putting that absolutely ridiculous statement aside, Watson has now written his own diet book, which details

* Watson decided to resign in November 2019, after I had already written my first draft. Rude. He has said he will continue to campaign for policy change, as well as promote his diet book, so I doubt we've seen the last of him here.

how he lost the weight. Just what the world needs, another diet book written by someone with no nutrition qualifications.

In an interview with the *Guardian*, Tom Watson claims that when he started reading the references in Aseem's book,* he found "they contradicted some of the public health advice that was available and the marketing messages, [particularly] about low-fat products". Which is more likely to be trustworthy: public health advice backed by decades of robust research, or a diet book designed to provoke and sell? Tough question that. Unfortunately, Aseem Malhotra and Tom Watson are now working together, with Watson attempting to challenge the government guidelines on how much fat we are advised to consume. He seems to think it should be higher, and that there shouldn't be a limit on saturated fat. He also seems to be under the impression that public health advice tells the public to eat a low-fat diet, which it definitely doesn't. He writes on his blog: "There are some powerful vested interests who will fight any public policy changes that reduce refined sugar from our diets and find it far more convenient just to blame saturated fats." I mean, sure the food industry isn't exactly excited about reformulation. But we have government guidelines that recommend strict limits on how much added sugar we consume, and we have a sugar tax on soft drinks, so that's not even close to true.

Hopefully the updated SACN report has done something to dissuade his misinformed campaign, but nevertheless his collaboration with Aseem and co is incredibly concerning. A fringe group on Twitter who encourage us to stop taking

---

* I too have read the references in Aseem's book, and most of the time the study he cites doesn't even back up his own arguments.

life-saving medication in favour of eating butter should not be entertained by MPs. And yet here we are.

What can you do?

I get it, policy isn't exactly the most interesting subject in the world. But it's an aspect of nutrition and health that doesn't get enough airtime, and it matters, because it shows that you as an individual can really make a difference, using social media as your weapon of choice.

Now obviously, someone like Jamie Oliver has millions of followers, which certainly helps when starting a conversation about a topic or creating a petition. But there are plenty of influencers out there who also have hundreds of thousands, if not millions, of followers who can have just as much power.

And while it certainly makes things easier, you don't even have to be a huge influencer to make a difference. Gina Martin currently has around 50,000 Instagram followers and 24,000 on Twitter, and she is responsible for making upskirting illegal in the UK. As of April 2019, offenders who take a photo under a person's clothes without their knowledge can now be arrested. If convicted, they will face up to two years in jail and may be placed on the sex offenders' register. Gina had no legal or political experience, no large sums of money, and not even close to millions of followers, but she changed the law in eighteen months. Along the way, she created a petition that was signed by over 110,000 people and created the hashtag #StopSkirtingTheIssue on social media to spread the word. It worked.

Another successful example is Nicola Thorp, a temp worker who was sent home from her job as a receptionist for wearing flat shoes rather than heels. She channelled her anger and frustration into an online petition calling for companies to be banned from instructing women to wear high heels at work, which was signed by more than 150,000 people. This petition led to a debate in Parliament as well as a joint report by the Petitions and Women and Equalities Committees, which found existing laws were not proving effective in preventing discrimination.

Social media is now one of the most powerful forms of activism and has real potential as a tool to effect change. There are several reasons why that is:

- Social media allows you to send more messages to more people, more quickly. It enables you to spread the word about a cause you believe in at a much faster rate and to a larger group of people than through traditional media. You can create a petition and have it reach thousands of people in mere hours, if not minutes.
- Social media has the potential to bring people fair and balanced news coverage, as news can come straight from the individual in their own words, rather than risk being twisted by media with an agenda. (Of course, this isn't always accurate, as misinformation can spread just as quickly as accurate information, while trolls can derail conversations and bully those they disagree with.)
- Social media gives the individual the power to call out injustices, inaccuracies and misrepresentations and brings about better understanding of other cultures and people. It gives ordinary people a voice far more easily than the traditional media.

- Social media enables people from all over the world to take part in important conversations and join together using hashtags. People from opposite sides of the globe who speak different languages can vocalise their common goals, and create awareness of issues right where people spend so much of their time. Social media meets people where they're at and then invites them to join in, to take something further through offline action.

- Social media is a more accessible way of activism for those who cannot leave their home. Those with certain disabilities, carers, and those with young children can get involved and make their voices heard, without being limited by their ability to get out to protests and so on. This allows for more diverse groups of people to be heard, and allows for a truer representation of the reality, not just privileged groups.

Now it's your turn

There's no doubt in my mind that social media can be an incredible way to reach and inspire you to get on board with a cause you believe in. As an influencer, I think you have to make a choice. Do you want your influence to focus on what people eat or what clothes they wear? Or do you also want to use that position to influence the decisions that people make that really have an impact? Something more fundamental that will make a difference?

When I say 'influencer' in this case, I don't just mean people with tens of thousands of followers, I mean anyone who has any influence over others, whether it's your 20 Twitter followers or

200 Facebook friends – it still counts. Social media offers you an unprecedented opportunity to use your voice and shout about something that matters to you, no matter how big or small. You can make a difference, but you have to have a clear message and strategy, and you have to put your heart behind it. And be prepared to fail, pick yourself up and try again.

Conclusion

HOW TO 'GRAM YOUR CAKE AND EAT IT TOO!

I find a lot of the media headlines around social media a little unfair. People are too quick to say that social media has turned us all into food-obsessed monsters, that food porn is causing us all to become fat, or that our food photos are signs of narcissism. This modern technology affects our food decisions and our relationship with food in both positive and negative ways. It can contribute to us feeling dissatisfied with our lives, or it can lead to connections that enrich our lives.

If you find yourself in the former category, if you're concerned that social media is making your health and wellbeing worse, know that there are things you can do to improve that. Telling people to avoid social media entirely is an unreasonable and unrealistic request. Once you're online it's difficult to let go.

Finding an online community can be a really positive thing, and there are loads of people out there using social media to promote amazing causes around food and health, such as niche food allergies and intolerance groups, body acceptance, and eating disorder recovery accounts. I understand that you're likely reading this because you're interested in food and health – great! But if your entire feed is nothing but 'clean eating' and #fitspo you may want to reassess. Follow those food and health accounts, but maybe also follow some cute puppies, travel photographers or houseplant accounts too.

On the flip side, if you're someone who posts food and health content online, please remember your own influence. Remember that every single one of your followers isn't just a number, they're a real person, and while you can post whatever the hell you want, be mindful of the effects your images can have on others. Sure, it may give you a sense of validation when you post a bikini picture that gets loads of likes, but what if that picture is making thousands of people feel shit about themselves? We can't be responsible for all extenuating circumstances or possibilities, but we can take others into consideration when we post. You may want to ask yourself: am I doing this for myself or for my followers? How will this make people feel? Is this more likely to be helpful or harmful?

Of course, the validation and praise you get online feels great. Anyone who says otherwise is probably lying. But social media shouldn't be the only source of our self-worth, it's far too fragile for that. Some external validation is unavoidable, but you don't want your self-worth to be heavily dependent on social media.

Stop comparing yourself

Comparing ourselves to others is inevitable, it is part of how human brains work. But while we cannot change the fact that we

Quiz: social comparison orientation scale

	STRONGLY DISAGREE	DISAGREE	NEITHER AGREE NOR DISAGREE	AGREE	STRONGLY AGREE
I often compare my accomplishments to others'	1	2	3	4	5
I pay a lot of attention to how I do things compared with others	1	2	3	4	5
I often compare how my loved ones are doing with how others are doing	1	2	3	4	5
I am not the type of person who compares often with others	5	4	3	2	1
If I want to find out how well I have done something, I compare with others	1	2	3	4	5
I often compare how I am doing socially (e.g., social skills, popularity) with other people	1	2	3	4	5

do sometimes engage in comparison, what we can do is change how we respond to it. To end this chapter, I offer some action plans for you, which I hope will help with exactly this.

Some of us do far more comparison than others, and knowing where you exist on that scale can be an interesting insight that can guide whether this may be something you need to work on. I'm sure you might have an intuitive idea, but who doesn't love a quiz to be sure?

Please remember this is not a diagnostic tool. Generally speaking, if your score is higher than 20, its likely that you are high in social comparison orientation. The lower your score, the less likely you are to engage in comparison.

If you score highly in social comparison orientation, it means you're probably someone who is more likely to engage in comparison because you're uncertain about yourself and want to try and fit in as much as possible. Yes, it's important to care a little about what others think, but not so much that it incapacitates you.

There are some areas in life where a little comparison is beneficial and normal. Of course, you'll compare your grades to your classmates, and you may look up to someone who you see as more successful than you, and that can drive your ambition. But when it comes to food and appearance, there's little evidence to suggest this is helpful.

The solution is not to be harsh on yourself when you find yourself engaging in upward social comparisons, nor is the solution to focus on downward comparisons either, as this still turns our bodies and food into a competition. What does seem to be beneficial is a shift in mindset from competition to compassion. Being kind and compassionate towards ourselves, and supporting ourselves, especially in times of distress, has been shown to improve our wellbeing and foster positive body image.

Action plan: Next time you're scrolling through social media and find yourself engaging in body or food comparisons (which are essentially the same thing, as our food choices are linked to our physical appearance), I would encourage you to do two things. First, show compassion and kindness towards your comparison target by giving them a compliment that isn't a comparison. Second, show compassion towards your-self, and remind yourself of how wonderful you are as a human. It might feel a little uncomfortable at first, but that's usually a sign that it's something that could be beneficial for you.

Action plan: The health and wellness space online is incredibly homogeneous. It seems as if so many of the most popular bloggers and influencers are straight, white, thin people. That doesn't represent the real world, so follow people who are a diverse range of body types, sizes, abilities, genders, identi-ties, ethnicities, and so on. Here are some of my favourites:

- @scarrednotscared
- @nerdabouttown
- @shisodelicious
- @kittehinfurs
- @lottielamour
- @jamie_windust
- @bodyposipanda
- @munroebergdorf
- @ihartericka
- @sittingpretty
- @dietitiananna

Own your identity

Although it's tempting to think we have complete power over how we are perceived online, we need to remember that we can never fully control other people's perceptions of ourselves. People will always make some judgement call about us based on what we post, and it's simply impossible to please everyone.

If you want to post your food pictures online, please go ahead! If you're finding it's a chore, maybe take a break for a while and reassess what your original intentions were.

Action plan: If you're finding yourself posting food pictures purely for other people, not for your own enjoyment, then challenge yourself by posting something that's exactly what you want to.

Eat mindfully

Distracted eating is often the norm for us – we have to watch something while we eat dinner, have to eat our lunch at our desk so it looks as though we're still working, and we scroll through our social media feeds while we eat our breakfast in the morning. This disconnects us from our food, leaving us less satisfied and less full.

Mindfulness is a learned skill that's linked to a number of positive outcomes. This quiz will help you see where you're at now, and where you can potentially improve to get to a more mindful place with food.

Quiz: mindful eating questionnaire

	NEVER	RARELY	SOMETIMES	OFTEN/ ALWAYS
I eat so quickly that I don't taste what I'm eating.	4	3	2	1
My thoughts tend to wander while I am eating.	4	3	2	1
I think about things I need to do while I am eating.	4	3	2	1
When I'm at a buffet, I tend to overeat.	4	3	2	1
When a restaurant portion is too large, I stop eating when I'm full.	1	2	3	4
When I'm eating one of my favourite foods, I don't recognise when I've had enough.	4	3	2	1
If it doesn't cost much more, I get the larger size food or drink regardless of how hungry I feel.	4	3	2	1
I snack without noticing that I'm eating.	4	3	2	1
I notice when there are subtle flavours in the foods I eat.	1	2	3	4

Add your total score. The higher the score the more of a mindful eater you are!

Action plan: If you scored low on the mindful eating quiz, my challenge to you is to have one meal a day where you are completely removed from all distractions. No phone, no screens at all, no audio. Just you and your food. If this is uncomfortable, think about why that might be. Are you worried you're not being productive enough? Are you afraid of missing something? Are you bored? If you can't go 15 or 20 minutes without some kind of distraction, that suggests something about your discomfort at spending time with your own thoughts that you might wish to address. Your productivity is actually likely to be higher overall if you take that time to focus on enjoying your food and refresh from work. There are plenty of other times you can watch or listen to something. With practice, I promise it gets easier.

Beware of food extremism

Holders of extreme views on social media don't tend to interact much and are more likely to engage with other people who hold similarly extreme views. This can lead to an echo-chamber effect that never challenges your ideas and views about the world. Exposure to a diverse range of viewpoints is crucial for developing well-informed humans who are also receptive to and tolerant of the ideas of others.

No matter how strong your views are, ensure your social media isn't an echo chamber of people who agree with you all the time. I follow people on Instagram who eat very differently to me, and I follow people on Twitter who have very different political, ideological and philosophical views from my own. This is important to me, to remind me on a regular basis that these people exist, and that they are human beings just like me. I think this is just as important in food as it is in areas such as politics, especially because food and nutrition can be such a divisive and heated topic.

Action plan: Follow people who eat in a variety of different ways, because not everyone eats the same way you do, nor should they.

Don't food shame

If you're posting about food online with a public profile, receiving shaming comments is, sadly, pretty much inevitable. While constructive criticism, or someone politely offering a correction to your work, is something that is vital and to be encouraged, there is a difference between this and outright aggressive shaming and trolling.

The only way to avoid any kind of criticism is to say nothing at all. There is a misconception that receiving criticism means you're doing something right, and while that's sometimes true, it's not always. Saying stupid and incorrect things also garners criticism.

Many of us (absolutely myself included) can respond to any kind of critique with defensiveness. I find it quite comforting to know that it's normal to have this immediate reaction. Social media is so instant that we want to reply straight away, simply because we can. My recommendation is simply not to do this. Close the app, take a few deep breaths, do something else, and come back to it with a clearer head. At that point, you can hopefully be more objective about which category the comment falls into: is it constructive or destructive? If it's the former, engage. If it's the latter, delete.

It's all very well to say 'Oh, don't take it personally', which tends to work just about as well as 'Don't worry!' (In other words: not at all.) Of course, we logically know not to take it personally but it does affect us, and that's OK. For me, under-standing why people post shaming comments and attacks has been instrumental in becoming less reactive. I think that under-standing helps support the statement of 'it's not about you, it's them', and gives it more weight, making it easier to believe. I want to make it clear that this doesn't justify those kinds of comments or make them OK, but simply makes them easier to manage when they do appear.

Action plan: Learn to differentiate between constructive criti-cism and shaming trolls. When you see a comment that hurts, don't react, take a moment to breathe and release some of that defensiveness, then come back to it when you're ready. If it's a shaming and unhelpful comment, you have every right to delete and/or block that person.

Say no to perfection

Remember, there is no such thing as a perfect diet. Those of us who tend to believe this idea of food perfection also tend to be more likely to be perfectionists. See where you fall on the per-fectionism scale with this quiz.

Quiz: Multidimensional perfectionism scale

SELF-ORIENTED PERFECTIONISM	STRONGLY DISAGREE	DISAGREE	NEITHER AGREE NOR DISAGREE	AGREE	STRONGLY AGREE
When I am working on something, I cannot relax until it is perfect.	1	2	3	4	5
One of my goals is to be perfect in everything I do.	1	2	3	4	5
It is very important that I am perfect in everything I attempt.	1	2	3	4	5
I strive to be the best at everything I do.	1	2	3	4	5
It makes me uneasy to see an error in my work.	1	2	3	4	5
I must work to my full potential at all times.	1	2	3	4	5
I set very high standards for myself.	1	2	3	4	5
I must always be successful at school or work.	1	2	3	4	5

SOCIALLY PRESCRIBED PERFECTIONISM	STRONGLY DISAGREE	DISAGREE	NEITHER AGREE NOR DISAGREE	AGREE	STRONGLY AGREE
I find it difficult to meet others' expectations of me.	1	2	3	4	5
Those around me don't accept that I can make mistakes too.	1	2	3	4	5
The people around me expect me to succeed at everything I do.	1	2	3	4	5
Others won't like me if I don't excel at everything.	1	2	3	4	5
Success means that I must work even harder to please others.	1	2	3	4	5
I feel that people are too demanding of me.	1	2	3	4	5
Although they may not say it, other people get very upset with me when I slip up.	1	2	3	4	5
My parents expect(ed) me to excel in all aspects of my life.	1	2	3	4	5
People expect more from me than I am capable of giving.	1	2	3	4	5

Add up your total score for each measure. The multidimensional perfectionism scale is not a clinical measure so there is not a clinical cut-off score, but the higher you score on each scale, the more unhealthy your perfectionistic attitudes and behaviours may be.

One of the key ways perfectionism can manifest in relation to food is through orthorexia (see pages 146–8). If you think you, or someone you know, is struggling with orthorexia, please do reach out. It can be hard to find professional help, and your doctor may not yet be aware of what orthorexia is (although that is thankfully slowly changing), but you deserve to be supported and helped in your recovery. You deserve to have a happy, healthy relationship with food.

As a psychologist, Kimberley Wilson often helps clients navigate social media: "I am big on understanding the meaning of a behaviour, so I'll want to understand the function and nature of the social media use. When are they using it? Is it a kind of self-harm? Does their use illustrate an ambivalence about recovery? I encourage people to take more responsibility for the information they consume; to not just passively absorb whatever the algorithm serves up. Unfollow accounts they *know* are undermining recovery. Follow accounts that offer an inclusive view of bodies and health. In fact, I will often ask them why they are looking at other people's bodies at all! It's actually a strange kind of voyeurism that brings no value to your life. I like the idea of curating your social media feed as you would a magazine. Would you buy a magazine that was just page after page of semi-naked people standing around in the gym? Most people wouldn't. So instead create your own magazine: recipes, travel, politics, literature, current affairs, science, comedy. Choose to be informed and entertained, not undermined. Be more mindful about the information you habitually consume."

Action plan: Follow accounts that don't just post the perfect, happy, smiley pictures, and find people who actively share their ups and downs, their food fails, and how there's no such thing as a perfect diet.

Action plan: Be imperfect online. Maybe start small, with a recipe fail or a 'less-than-perfect' image of yourself where you're in the moment and having an amazing time. Notice how nothing bad happens! As a recovering perfectionist myself, what I've found most helpful has been mentally replacing the word 'perfect' with 'good enough'.

Take care of your health

If you find that social media is making you feel worse about yourself, re-examine who you follow. Take some time away and discuss your experiences online with a mental health professional who can help.

It's absolutely possible to obtain more benefits than downsides from social media. One of the crucial ways we can do this is by making sure we're not spending too much time online, and by engaging with people online rather than simply just scrolling. Remember that sense of community on social media can be so important and can actually improve our overall wellbeing. Find people online who you connect with and have meaningful conversations with them.

Also, be very sceptical of health information online. Check it's coming from reputable sources who have qualifications and evidence to back them up. There is so much health misinformation out there, often coming from people with no expertise in the area they're so keen to shout about.

Action plan: Use phone settings or apps to set limits on your time online. Most smartphones will now track your screen time for you, and you might be shocked at how high it is. Set yourself a daily limit for your social media apps. My recommendation: start by taking your current social media screen time and rounding down to the nearest hour. When you reach your limit, your phone will prevent you from being able to access those apps without a manual override. Of course, you can simply say 'give me another 15 minutes', but it's an extra step that forces you to consider whether you actually need to check Facebook again, or if you're simply doing it automatically out of habit or boredom.

What keeps you on social media?

There are a lot of negative health implications of social media, particularly in regard to our mental health, so I wanted to find out from some of the people I interviewed what keeps them on social media, and how they ensure social media is a safe and fun place for them. Their answers, combined with my own, hopefully provide a positive conclusion. Here are some of the patterns in their answers.

Connection

Becky Excell: "I've met some amazing humans who I hope will

be friends for life. I would never have met them without my blog and social media."

Tally Rye: "Social media has brought me friendships and connection, it's given me a voice and a platform, and it's given me a chance to listen to other people's stories."

P: "It blows my mind that we have this access to other people in a way that we've never known before, people outside of our bubble and our understanding of the world. I think it's really good for connecting with people whose thoughts or life experiences differ from yours, as well as people who can relate to your experiences. That is why the online skin community exists, it's because a lot of people don't see their skin represented around them and there's something very healing about finding this solidarity with other people, and hearing them voice what you're also thinking."

Sharing of information and expertise

Charlotte Stirling-Reed: "Everyone probably says this... but what keeps me online are the messages I get from followers saying that they were incredibly anxious about weaning until they found my page and now they love feeding their baby and watching them explore new foods. Giving confidence!"

Kimberley Wilson: "As a psychologist I have a huge amount of access to information that can help people to live happier, more satisfying lives, and years of experience implementing that knowledge. It doesn't make sense to me that that information isn't more widely available to the public. I use my platform to disseminate this information as widely as possible. I see it as part of my professional role. I also learn from professionals in other fields and have met many friends and colleagues through social media."

Inspiration and learning

Becky Excell: "I love using social media for recipe inspiration; Instagram is so visual and always gives me great ideas."

Maxine Ali: "I stay because social media can be an incredible think tank, for critical, intelligent and innovative ideas from changemakers that spark incredible transformations in the world. Like it or not, social media is at the centre of information-sharing, and I wouldn't want to miss out on all those opportunities to learn."

P: "Having access to experts and people who know what they're talking about is amazing. We wouldn't have the kind of conversations we're able to have without experts sharing their knowledge and expertise online. Hearing an expert say something like 'dairy doesn't cause acne' feels like permission and feels so reassuring." (I agree, when expertise is used appropriately and that responsibility is not abused online, it's a wonderful thing.)

Creative expression

Izy Hossack: "Sometimes I would like to quit Instagram, but it's my portfolio, and as long as people are around and using social media, I'll be posting."

Sara Kiyo Popowa: "Deleting my account, what a nightmare haha! Well... to me, my account is first and foremost a space for creative expression and exploration, and a place to get my views and messages out to a fair amount of people. Until something better comes along I'm definitely sticking to this! Any artist needs an audience, to be witnessed, whether it is by your closest family or millions of people. Exhibiting one's work, one's expression – whether it is visual, writing, food concepts or the whole experience of being alive and developing one's beliefs and convictions – to an audience who enable you to develop as a person and as an artist is just priceless. I used to do other types of artwork before social media and never did I experience such a response as I have now. It's just the right time in my life and the right time to express the things I want to express."

I agree with all of these, and they're all reasons I choose to stay on social media as well. I've met so many of my close friends through Instagram, it's a great way to share the knowledge and experience I've gained in the field of nutrition with a wide group of people, I learn so much from other professionals I follow, and it's a wonderful creative outlet.

How do you ensure that social media is a safe space?

You can never guarantee that going online is going to be a safe or enjoyable experience, but that doesn't mean your experience has to feel totally out of your hands. There are tricks and tools you can put into place to regain some control over your online experience, whether emotional or practical. Once again, I asked some of the wonderful experts and individuals I interviewed for this book to share how they protect themselves and set boundaries online, in the hope that our collective wisdom will be more useful.

Setting limits

Izy Hossack: "I have a daily time limit on my social media, and while I can override it it's an extra step, so it makes me pause and think. I also notice that when I actually interact with people it becomes a positive experience, whereas when I just mindlessly scroll through, I feel like I haven't gained anything from it at all."

P: "I limit my time online to avoid getting too absorbed in it and overwhelmed by it all."

Charlotte Stirling-Reed: "I'm learning this too! I have to have my social media boundaries – I know I'm much better, more motivated and supportive when I do this – but I'm not always good at sticking to them. One thing I really try to do is stay off for the majority of the weekend (I post Saturday a.m. and then don't go on much until Raffy is asleep or the weekend is over), and try to spend real time with friends and family and just be 'in the moment'."

Privacy

Maxine: "I really rate having a private account on social media platforms, one that is just for me and perhaps a few select people I give permission to let in. In this space, there's no pressure to perform the 'best' version of me, to paint a perfect life or prove my worth and success. It's purely about sharing stories and staying connected, with boundaries I can command to best protect me."

Carmen Huter: "I set boundaries for myself in terms of the content I share and the ways I attach myself to something so intangible. This is a big reason as to why I started creating my photo workshops, as they allow me to share everything I do on social media offline and in real-time with real people in front of me."

Being firm

P: "I use the block button liberally and try not to feel guilty about it. I also avoid using certain hashtags that I know attract trolls."

Sasha:* "I am far more sceptical of wild claims being made and do my research on who people are and what their qualifications are before I consider their advice as being worthwhile."

Cassidy: "When I see a post now I question the source. Is this a person that is just focused on their image and has no background in health? Is this a realistic image of how life is? I avoid any accounts that do not provide a realistic view of life mostly, and stick with those that inspire me instead."

Choose who you follow

Tally Rye: "My consumption of social media has changed massively from always looking at inspirational content to educational content, so social media is a totally different experience. Where I used to just follow health and fitness stuff, now I follow Broadway people, fashion, comedy... just getting out of my bubble."

Michelle Elman: "I am very selective about who I follow and I am very conscious of when it is time to step away from social media and turn my phone off."

* name changed.

Karl:* "I unfollowed all the people who made me feel like shit and replaced them with people who don't."

Rebecca: "I have regular 'culls' of those who I follow in order to make sure that I only see messages that I see to be beneficial to my mental health. I also now believe myself to be much better at identifying false claims and take messages from those without qualifications with a pinch of salt."

Kindness and compassion

P: "I remind myself that anyone who leaves nasty, hateful comments is not a happy person."

Becky Excell: "When you work for yourself there's this constant pressure, you have no salary, no holiday pay etc., so you feel like you must keep working. But I feel like if I could allow myself a little more time off, away from my phone completely, that would help a lot. It's a work in progress!"

Tally Rye: "I give myself full permission to post whenever I want. There is no pressure to post."

Rachel Hugh: "It's a tough thing to do, but set yourself limits, remember you are one person behind the screen talking to thousands of followers at any one time. One negative comment can set you in a tailspin for the rest of your day, so never forget that one person doesn't speak for the majority; always remember that you are human with real emotions, it's totally OK to step away when it gets too much."

Kimberley Wilson: "All I can do is act with integrity and kindness, which I try to do. Everything else is out of my hands."

* name changed.

*

So many wise words! I hope that this inspires you to assess your own boundaries online, whether they're related to time spent online, over-sharing, dealing with hateful comments, or simply ensuring that your feed lifts you up rather than drags you down.

A final few bites of wisdom

Overall, social media has had a significant impact on how we eat: it's changing *what* we choose to eat, *how* we eat, and why we choose the foods we do; it's contributed to more and more extreme ideas about food, led to an explosion of misinformation, provided an easy platform for us to judge and shame one another, and added extra pressure to be perfect. But social media is also opening up new avenues for recipe inspiration, sharing of health expertise, and food communities.

Social media has drastically changed the way we interact with the food industry and the restaurant industry. The focus has shifted from a gastronomic experience to an aesthetic one, where eating with our eyes through our phone screens sometimes matters more than how the food tastes. A brand or a restaurant without a social media presence is now something to be wary of (unless you're in Italy, of course).

Social media is even now influencing public health, both in positive encouraging ways, and through frightening fringe influences that would likely otherwise not have accumulated so much power.

Through all this, there are individuals using their influence on these maligned platforms to do good, to create communities, promote noble causes and counter misinformation.

In the end, these social media platforms are simply tools. There's no way to embrace the immense good such tools can do without learning to live with, and mitigate, their downsides. They're a package deal.

Social media cannot be undone. It's here now and it's here to stay. These platforms get an incredibly bad rep, and in some cases, they really deserve it. But not completely. Not always. If I've shown you anything, it's that you hold in your hand a tool with which to do either some good or some harm. Most likely it's a bit of both. That's an incredible power - use it wisely!

Bibliography/Resources

Introduction

p. 2   '...linked with higher self-esteem': Burrow, A. L., & Rainone, N. (2017). How many likes did I get?: Purpose moderates links between positive social media feedback and self-esteem. *Journal of Experimental Social Psychology*, *69*, 232–236.

p. 2   'In a survey in 2017...': New Statesman survey. https://www. newstatesman.com/science-tech/social-media/2017/01/both-hugely-uplifting-and-depressing-how-do-social-media-likes

p. 3   'Categorized by age...': https://www.emarketer.com/Chart/US-Social-Media-Users-by-Generation-2019-of-population/226029

p. 3   '...2 out of 5 minutes we spend online': GlobalWebIndex. (2016). GWI Social: GlobalWebIndex's quarterly report on the latest trends in social networking. Retrieved from http://blog. globalwebindex.net/chart-of-the-day/social-media-captures-30-ofonline-time/

p. 3   '...60% feel they use their phone too much': http://www.deloitte. co.uk/mobileuk/#uk-excessive-phone-or-smartphone-usage-by-age-group /Deloitte 2018 survey in general (link available soon).

p. 4   '158 minutes per day on social media...': Emarsys, 2019 https://www.emarsys.com/resources/blog/top-5-social-media-predictions-2019/

p. 4   '...lose access to their phone or computer': McCann The Truth About Youth survey. https://www.ceap.org.ph/upload/download/20135/2164130287_1.pdf

p. 4   '...check their phone during the night': http://www.deloitte. co.uk/mobileuk/#uk-effects-of-excessive-smartphone-usage

p. 5   Sean Parker interview: https://www.axios.com/sean-parker-unloads-on-facebook-god-only-knows-what-its-doing-to-our-childrens-brains-1513306792-f855e7b4-4e99-4d60-8d51-2775559c2671.html

p. 6   "little bits of positivity": https://www.theguardian.com/technology/2017/oct/05/smartphone-addiction-silicon-valley-dystopia

p. 6   Eyal, N. (2014). *Hooked: How to Build Habit-Forming Products*, Penguin.

p. 12   '63% of 13–32-year-olds': YPulse survey from 2015. https://www.ypulse.com/article/2015/05/18/foodporn-the-growing-influence-of-social-food/

p. 12   '84% of daily pinners...': Ahalogy. 2016 Pinterest Media Consumption Study. https://micwatching.files.wordpress.com/2016/10/8385c-ahalogypinterestmediaconsumptionstudy2016.pdf

p. 13   'The term 'food porn' goes back to 1979': https://www.entrepreneur.com/article/295126

p. 14   'An examination of 10 million Instagram posts...': #foodporn around the world: Mejova, Y., Abbar, S., & Haddadi, H. (2016). Fetishizing food in digital age: #foodporn around the world. In *Tenth International AAAI Conference on Web and Social Media*.

p. 17   "The history of any nation's diet is the history of the nation itself...": Bell, D. and Valentine, G. (1997). *Consuming Geographies: We Are Where We Eat*. Routledge. (ebook 2013)

p. 18   'Research back in the 1980s...': Sadalla, E., & Burroughs, J. (1981). Profiles in Eating: Sexy vegetarians and other diet-based social stereotypes. *Psychology today*, 15(10), 51.

p. 19   '...rate individuals based on their diets': Steim, R. I. and Nemeroff, C. J. (1995). Moral overtones of food: judgments of others based on what they eat'. *Personality and Social Psychology Bulletin*, (21): 480–90.

p. 19   'Other studies reported a more varied picture...'. Summary here: Vartanian, L. R., Herman, C. P., & Polivy, J. (2007). Consumption stereotypes and impression management: How you are what you eat. *Appetite*, 48(3), 265–277.

p. 23   '...a social condition that has been dubbed 'strange familiarity'':

Familiar stranger: Senft, T. M. (2013). Microcelebrity and the branded self. *A companion to new media dynamics*, 346–354.

p. 26   '...98% of these are upward social comparisons': Jan, M., Soomro, S., & Ahmad, N. (2017). Impact of social media on self-esteem.

p. 26   'frequent Facebook users believe...': Vogel, E. A., Rose, J. P., Roberts, L. R., & Eckles, K. (2014). Social comparison, social media, and self-esteem. *Psychology of Popular Media Culture*, *3*(4), 206.

p. 27   '90% of Americans aged 18–24 years have indicated...: PwC Health Research Institute Social Media "Likes" Healthcare: From Marketing to Social Business. 2012. http://download.pwc.com/ie/pubs/2012_social_media_likes_healthcare.pdf.

p. 28   The Great American Search for Healthcare Information: https://www.webershandwick.com/news/the-great-american-search-for-healthcare-information/

p. 28   "had the potential to harm cancer patients if the advice provided was followed": Ernst, E., Schmidt, K. (2002). 'Alternative' cancer cures via the Internet? *British Journal of Cancer*, (87); 479–80

p. 28   '...2.5 times more likely to die within five years': Johnson, S. B., Park, H. S., Gross, C. P., & Yu, J. B. (2017). Use of alternative medicine for cancer and its impact on survival. *JNCI: Journal of the National Cancer Institute*, *110*(1), 121–124.

p. 28   'accuracy of information about coeliac disease...': England, C. Y., & Nicholls, A. M. (2004). Advice available on the Internet for people with coeliac disease: an evaluation of the quality of websites. *Journal of human nutrition and dietetics*, *17*(6), 547–559.

Chapter 1

p. 34   '...consistent effect on food choice.': Robinson, E., Thomas, J., Aveyard, P., & Higgs, S. (2014). What everyone else is eating: a systematic review and meta-analysis of the effect of informational eating norms on eating behavior. *Journal of the Academy of Nutrition and Dietetics*, *114*(3), 414–429.

p. 34   '...the wrappers were evidence enough.': Prinsen, S., de Ridder,

D. T. and de Vet, E. (2013). Eating by example. Effects of environmental cues on dietary decisions. *Appetite*, 70: 1–5.

p. 34   '...regardless of body size, gender, weight, hunger or age': Cruwys, T., Bevelander, K. E., & Hermans, R. C. (2015). Social modeling of eating: A review of when and why social influence affects food intake and choice. *Appetite*, *86*, 3–18.

p. 36   '...claimed afterwards that they were hungry': Bevelander, K. E., Anschütz, D. J., Creemers, D. H., Kleinjan, M., & Engels, R. C. (2013). The role of explicit and implicit self-esteem in peer modeling of palatable food intake: a study on social media interaction among youngsters. *PloS one*, *8*(8), e72481.

p. 41   '...rise of Instagram with the growth of veganism': https://www.independent.co.uk/life-style/food-and-drink/veganism-rise-uk-why-instagram-mainstream-plant-based-diet-vegans-popularity-a8296426.html

p. 42   '...a recent study about pizza': Polivy, J., Herman, C. P., & Deo, R. (2010). Getting a bigger slice of the pie. Effects on eating and emotion in restrained and unrestrained eaters. *Appetite*, *55*(3), 426–430.

p. 44   '...eat more pizza and enjoy it more too.': Polivy, J., & Pliner, P. (2015). "She got more than me". Social comparison and the social context of eating. *Appetite*, *86*, 88–95.

p. 46   'Research shows that high SCO individuals...': Vogel, E. A., Rose, J. P., Okdie, B. M., Eckles, K., & Franz, B. (2015). Who compares and despairs? The effect of social comparison orientation on social media use and its outcomes. *Personality and Individual Differences*, *86*, 249–256.

p. 52   '...understanding how these stereotypes may affect our eating behaviour' (and rest of this section): Vartanian, L. R., Herman, C. P., & Polivy, J. (2007). Consumption stereotypes and impression management: How you are what you eat. *Appetite*, *48*(3), 265–277.

p. 55   '...all light up in imaging studies.': van Meer, F., van der Laan, L. N., Adan, R. A., Viergever, M. A., & Smeets, P. A. (2015). What you see is what you eat: an ALE meta-analysis of the neural correlates of food viewing in children and adolescents. *Neuroimage*, *104*, 35–43.

p. 56   'influence their appetite and their food choices.': Vaterlaus, J. M., Patten, E. V., Roche, C., & Young, J. A. (2015). # Gettinghealthy:

The perceived influence of social media on young adult health behaviors. *Computers in Human Behavior, 45*, 151–157.

Chapter 2

p. 59 'The term 'phubbing' defines the act...': Chotpitayasunondh, V., & Douglas, K. M. (2016). How "phubbing" becomes the norm: The antecedents and consequences of snubbing via smartphone. *Computers in Human Behavior, 63*, 9–18.

p. 60 '...have fuelled obsessive and unhealthy behaviour.': E.g. https://time.com/5066561/health-data-tracking-obsession/

p. 61 'working people in Singapore were randomly assigned...': Finkelstein, E. A., Haaland, B. A., Bilger, M., Sahasranaman, A., Sloan, R. A., Nang, E. E. K., & Evenson, K. R. (2016). Effectiveness of activity trackers with and without incentives to increase physical activity (TRIPPA): a randomised controlled trial. *The lancet Diabetes & endocrinology, 4*(12), 983–995.

p. 62 '...at the expense of pleasure and creativity.': Etkin, J. (2016). The hidden cost of personal quantification. *Journal of Consumer Research, 42*(6), 967–984.

p. 63 '...eating disorder symptoms among college students.': Simpson, C. C., & Mazzeo, S. E. (2017). Calorie counting and fitness tracking technology: Associations with eating disorder symptomatology. *Eating behaviors, 26*, 89–92.

p. 63 'survey of female Fitbit users undertaken in 2016...': https://edition.cnn.com/2016/09/01/health/dark-side-of-fitness-trackers/index.html

p. 64 'Instagram is a commonly used tool...': Chung, C. F., Agapie, E., Schroeder, J., Mishra, S., Fogarty, J., & Munson, S. A. (2017, May). When personal tracking becomes social: Examining the use of Instagram for healthy eating. In *Proceedings of the 2017 CHI Conference on Human Factors in Computing Systems* (pp. 1674–1687). ACM.

p. 70 'more than a third of respondents to a UK survey...': https://www.deloitte.co.uk/mobileuk2017/assets/img/download/global-mobile-consumer-survey-2017_uk-cut.pdf

p. 70   '...71% more mac and cheese while watching tv.': Blass, E. M., Anderson, D. R., Kirkorian, H. L., Pempek, T. A., Price, I., & Koleini, M. F. (2006). On the road to obesity: Television viewing increases intake of high-density foods. *Physiology & behavior*, *88*(4–5), 597–604.

p. 71   '...eat more than we may need to.': Robinson, E., Aveyard, P., Daley, A., Jolly, K., Lewis, A., Lycett, D., & Higgs, S. (2013). Eating attentively: a systematic review and meta-analysis of the effect of food intake memory and awareness on eating. *The American journal of clinical nutrition*, *97*(4), 728–742.

p. 72   '...included three linked studies.': Coary, S., & Poor, M. (2016). How consumer-generated images shape important consumption outcomes in the food domain. *Journal of Consumer Marketing*, *33*(1), 1–8.

p. 73   'In one experiment, people were given a chocolate bar...': Vohs, K. D., Wang, Y., Gino, F., & Norton, M. I. (2013). Rituals enhance consumption. *Psychological Science*, *24*(9), 1714–1721.

p. 76   ""When I first started my account, yes, I was eating everything.".: From 'Food and Wine' interview: https://www.foodandwine.com/news/questions-food-instagram-influencers-answered

pp. 77–78   From Maxine quotes: Lavis, A. (2017). Food porn, pro-anorexia and the viscerality of virtual affect: Exploring eating in cyberspace. *Geoforum*, *84*, 198–205.
Mejova, Y., Abbar, S., & Haddadi, H. (2016, March). Fetishizing food in digital age:# foodporn around the world. In *Tenth International AAAI Conference on Web and Social Media*.
Lupton, D. (2017). Vitalities and visceralities: Alternative body/food politics in new digital media. *Alternative food politics: from the margins to the mainstream*.

Chapter 3

p. 88   '...ten threats to global health in 2019': https://www.who.int/emergencies/ten-threats-to-global-health-in-2019

p. 89   '...killed while trying to take selfies.': https://en.wikipedia.org/wiki/List_of_selfie-related_injuries_and_deaths

p. 90   '...hold similarly extreme views.': Bright, J. (2017). Explaining the emergence of echo chambers on social media: the role of ideology and extremism. *Available at SSRN 2839728*.

p. 90   '...perceived as credible, trustworthy and reliable.': Chu, S. C., & Kim, Y. (2011). Determinants of consumer engagement in electronic word-of-mouth (eWOM) in social networking sites. *International journal of Advertising*, *30*(1), 47–75.

p. 91   'In an article for the *New York Times* in 2018...': https://www.nytimes.com/2018/03/10/opinion/sunday/youtube-politics-radical.html

p. 103 '...more likely to hold sexist views.': Allcorn, A., & Ogletree, S. M. (2018). Linked oppression: Connecting animal and gender attitudes. *Feminism & Psychology*, *28*(4), 457–469.

p. 108 '...a 2015 interview for the *Guardian*': https://www.theguardian.com/lifeandstyle/2015/feb/15/truth-about-miracle-foods-chia-seeds-coconut-oil

Chapter 4

p. 111 'They were having a field day.': https://www.buzzfeednews.com/article/tanyachen/famous-vegan-youtuber-rawvana-allegedly-caught-eating-fish

p. 112 '..." a huge identity crisis" to eat animal products again.': https://www.buzzfeednews.com/article/stephaniemcneal/vegan-youtuber-eats-raw-eggs-salmon

p. 115 'You Did Not Eat That': https://www.mic.com/articles/89749/there-s-a-disturbing-new-food-shaming-trend-targeting-women-on-instagram

p. 116 "...woman eating succulent, dripping, greasy, comforting food?": https://www.nytimes.com/2011/02/16/dining/16interview.html?pagewanted=all&_r=0

p. 118 'In one interesting study on organic food...': Eskine, K. J. (2013). Wholesome foods and wholesome morals? Organic foods reduce prosocial behavior and harshen moral judgments. *Social Psychological and Personality Science*, *4*(2), 251–254.

p. 119 "...our own perceived shaming deficiency.": Brown, Brené (2015). *Daring Greatly: How the Courage to Be Vulnerable Transforms the Way We Live, Love, Parent, and Lead*, Penguin.

p. 127 "...simply wrong from a scientific one.": https://www.insider.com/dermatologist-shut-down-acne-food-shaming-instagram-2018-7

Chapter 5

p. 141 '...referred to as socially prescribed perfectionism.': Hewitt, P. L., & Flett, G. L. (1991). Perfectionism in the self and social contexts: conceptualization, assessment, and association with psychopathology. *Journal of personality and social psychology*, *60*(3), 456.

p. 142 '...by 33% – between 1989 and 2016.': Curran, T., & Hill, A. P. (2019). Perfectionism is increasing over time: A meta-analysis of birth cohort differences from 1989 to 2016. *Psychological Bulletin*, *145*(4), 410.

p. 144 '...reaches a point where it's crippling.': Hewitt, P. L., & Flett, G. L. (1991). Perfectionism in the self and social contexts: conceptualization, assessment, and association with psycho-pathology. *Journal of personality and social psychology*, *60*(3), 456.

p. 146 '...a strong desire to control health status.': Hanganu-Bresch, C. (2019). Orthorexia: eating right in the context of healthism. *Medical humanities*, medhum-2019.

p. 149 '...added pressure to be the perfect mum'. Data from London-based mothers' meet-up app Mush, discussed here: https://www.standard.co.uk/lifestyle/london-life/perfect-lives-of-instamums-are-making-london-mothers-feel-inadaquate-a3468426.html

p. 150 '...may contribute to parenting stress in mothers.': Padoa, T., Berle, D., & Roberts, L. (2018). Comparative social media use and the mental health of mothers with high levels of perfectionism. *Journal of Social and Clinical Psychology*, *37*(7), 514–535.

p. 150 "...from a professional when they need it the most.": https://www.vice.com/en_us/article/kzjm7e/mom-culture-instagram-mental-health

p. 155 Dimly Lit Meals for One: https://dimlylitmealsforone.tumblr.com

BIBLIOGRAPHY/RESOURCES   319

p. 155 Sad Desk Lunch: https://saddesklunch.com/
p. 155 Cooking for bae: https://www.instagram.com/cookingforbae/

Chapter 6

p. 160 '...poorer physical health and life satisfaction.': Shakya, H. B., & Christakis, N. A. (2017). Association of Facebook use with compromised well-being: A longitudinal study. *American journal of epidemiology, 185*(3), 203–211.

p. 161 '...depression and anxiety are substantially higher.': Primack, B. A., Shensa, A., Escobar-Viera, C. G., Barrett, E. L., Sidani, J. E., Colditz, J. B., & James, A. E. (2017). Use of multiple social media platforms and symptoms of depression and anxiety: A nationally-representative study among US young adults. *Computers in human behavior, 69*, 1–9.

p. 161 '...the lower your self-esteem may sink.': Jan, M., Soomro, S., & Ahmad, N. (2017). Impact of social media on self-esteem. *European Scientific Journal, 13*, 329–341.
and
Vogel, E. A., Rose, J. P., Roberts, L. R., & Eckles, K. (2014). Social comparison, social media, and self-esteem. *Psychology of Popular Media Culture, 3*(4), 206.

p. 162 '...associated with self-esteem, but only temporarily.': Burrow, A. L., & Rainone, N. (2017). How many likes did I get?: Purpose moderates links between positive social media feedback and self-esteem. *Journal of Experimental Social Psychology, 69*, 232–236.

p. 163 '...your body and eating over a year ahead.': Holland, G., & Tiggemann, M. (2016). A systematic review of the impact of the use of social networking sites on body image and disordered eating outcomes. *Body image, 17*, 100–110.

p. 164 '...more muscular than those in women's magazines.': Frederick, D. A., Fessler, D. M., & Haselton, M. G. (2005). Do representations of male muscularity differ in men's and women's magazines?. *Body Image, 2*(1), 81–86.

p. 164 '...excessive exercise, and steroid use among men.': Hobza, C.

L., Walker, K. E., Yakushko, O., & Peugh, J. L. (2007). What about men? Social comparison and the effects of media images on body and self-esteem. *Psychology of men & masculinity*, 8(3), 161.

p. 164   'Transgender and gender non-conforming (TGNC) individuals...': Carmel, T. C., & Erickson-Schroth, L. (2016). Mental health and the transgender population. Psychiatric Annals, 46(6), 346–349.

p. 165   '...can help foster resilience to discrimination.': Pflum, S. R., Testa, R. J., Balsam, K. F., Goldblum, P. B., & Bongar, B. (2015). Social support, trans community connectedness, and mental health symptoms among transgender and gender nonconforming adults. *Psychology of sexual orientation and gender diversity*, 2(3), 281.

p. 166   'This theory also helps to explain why gay...': Chmielewski, J. F., & Yost, M. R. (2013). Psychosocial influences on bisexual women's body image: Negotiating gender and sexuality. *Psychology of Women Quarterly*, 37(2), 224–241.

p. 174   "The way I saw it I had two choices.": http://www.dolly.com.au/lifestyle/im-healing-myself-from-cancer-naturally-9850

p. 176   '...entire food groups, including sugar.': https://www.thetimes.co.uk/article/teens-at-risk-from-clean-eating-logtd9vc8

p. 176   '...since the rise of social media.': Curran, T., & Hill, A. P. (2019). Perfectionism is increasing over time: A meta-analysis of birth cohort differences from 1989 to 2016. *Psychological Bulletin*, 145(4), 410.

p. 177   '...which is in itself a consumption stereotype.': Vartanian, L. R., Herman, C. P., & Polivy, J. (2007). Consumption stereotypes and impression management: How you are what you eat. *Appetite*, 48(3), 265–277.

p. 179   '...attempting to gain admiration and respect from others.': Hellmann, E. (2016). Keeping up appearances: perfectionism and perfectionistic self-presentation on social media. *DePauw University*.

p. 179   "every parent's and teacher's idea of perfection": Bruch, H. (2001). The golden cage: The enigma of anorexia nervosa. Harvard University Press.

p. 180   'Around 70% of people with anorexia score highly...': Bardone-
         Cone, A. M., Wonderlich, S. A., Frost, R. O., Bulik, C. M.,
         Mitchell, J. E., Uppala, S., & Simonich, H. (2007). Perfectionism
         and eating disorders: Current status and future directions.
         Clinical psychology review, *27*(3), 384–405.

p. 180   '...strongest association with eating disorders.': Bulik, C. M.,
         Tozzi, F., Anderson, C., Mazzeo, S. E., Aggen, S., & Sullivan, P. F.
         (2003). The relation between eating disorders and components of
         perfectionism. *American Journal of Psychiatry*, *160*(2), 366–368.

p. 181   'In a meta-analysis published in 2017...': Smith, M. M., Sherry,
         S. B., Chen, S., Saklofske, D. H., Mushquash, C., Flett, G. L.,
         & Hewitt, P. L. (2018). The perniciousness of perfectionism: A
         meta-analytic review of the perfectionism–suicide relationship.
         Journal of Personality, *86*(3), 522–542.

p. 183   '...shame avoidance behaviour, and biological mechanisms.':
         Dolezal, L., & Lyons, B. (2017). Health-related shame: an affective
         determinant of health?. *Medical Humanities*, *43*(4), 257–263.

p. 185   '...leading to a shame spiral that's difficult to escape from.':
         Orth, U., Berking, M., & Burkhardt, S. (2006). Self-conscious
         emotions and depression: Rumination explains why shame
         but not guilt is maladaptive. *Personality and social psychology
         bulletin*, *32*(12), 1608–1619.

p. 186   '...sedentary behaviour by encouraging more screen time.':
         Leung, L., & Lee, P. S. (2005). Multiple determinants of life
         quality: The roles of Internet activities, use of new media, social
         support, and leisure activities. *Telematics and Informatics*, *22*(3),
         161–180.

p. 186   '...above 6–8 hours per day of total sitting.': Patterson, R.,
         McNamara, E., Tainio, M., de Sá, T. H., Smith, A. D., Sharp,
         S. J., ... & Wijndaele, K. (2018). Sedentary behaviour and risk
         of all-cause, cardiovascular and cancer mortality, and incident
         type 2 diabetes: a systematic review and dose response meta-
         analysis. *European Journal of Epidemiology*, 33: 811.

p. 186   'In one 2017 survey conducted in the UK...': http://www.
         deloitte.co.uk/mobileuk/#uk-effects-of-excessive-smartphone-
         usage

p. 187   '...depression and anxiety, and lower self-esteem.': Woods, H. C.,

& Scott, H. (2016). # Sleepyteens: Social media use in adolescence is associated with poor sleep quality, anxiety, depression and low self-esteem. *Journal of adolescence*, *51*, 41–49.

p. 187   '...that's a whole other scenario.': Oh, H. J., Ozkaya, E., & LaRose, R. (2014). How does online social networking enhance life satisfaction? The relationships among online supportive interaction, affect, perceived social support, sense of community, and life satisfaction. *Computers in Human Behavior*, *30*, 69–78.

Chapter 7

p. 191   'Surveys show that 73% of marketers...': https://buffer.com/state-of-social-2019

p. 192   '...recommend the brand to their friends and family.': https://www.lyfemarketing.com/blog/social-media-marketing-statistics/

p. 193   '...campaigns earn about $6.50 for each dollar spent...': https://digitalmarketinginstitute.com/en-us/blog/20-influencer-marketing-statistics-that-will-surprise-you

p. 204   "...either of the authorised health claims.": https://www.asa.org.uk/rulings/protein-world-ltd-a17-389142.html

p. 204   'In June 2019 the ASA partnered...': https://www.asa.org.uk/news/asa-itv-couple-up-to-help-love-islanders-use-ad.html
and
https://www.asa.org.uk/uploads/assets/uploaded/3af39c72-76e1-4a59-b2b47e81a034cd1d.pdf

p. 207   'Research with adults shows that a disclosure...': Coates, A. E., Hardman, C. A., Halford, J. C. G., Christiansen, P., & Boyland, E. J. (2019). The effect of influencer marketing of food and a "protective" advertising disclosure on children's food intake. *Pediatric obesity*, e12540.

p. 208   'Research shows that when children consume a greater quantity...': Coates, A. E., Hardman, C. A., Halford, J. C., Christiansen, P., & Boyland, E. J. (2019). Social Media Influencer Marketing and Children's Food Intake: A Randomized Trial. *Pediatrics*, *143*(4), e20182554.

p. 209 '...social media influencers are masters of this.': Glucksman, M. (2017). The rise of social media influencer marketing on lifestyle branding: A case study of Lucie Fink. *Elon Journal of Undergraduate Research in Communications*, 8(2), 77–87.

Chapter 8

p. 213 'More than half of UK Twitter users log on...': https://blog.twitter.com/en_gb/a/en-gb/2014/foodie-tweets-10-facts-about-twitter-restaurants-and-food.html

p. 214 'According to research by the restaurant chain Zizzi...': https://www.independent.co.uk/life-style/food-and-drink/millenials-restaurant-how-choose-instagram-social-media-where-eat-a7677786.html

p. 214 '71% of customers say they're more likely to recommend...': https://www.prnewswire.com/news-releases/new-study-reveals-that-todays-consumers-demand-customer-service-via-social-media-175781781.html

p. 216 '...they make up for in likes and comments.': https://www.eater.com/2017/7/6/15925940/instagram-influencers-cronuts-milkshakes-burgers

p. 218 'Grind, the popular London cafe-bar chain...': https://www.bbc.co.uk/news/uk-england-london-42012732

p. 220 '...Heston Blumenthal, has a no-flash policy.': https://www.telegraph.co.uk/foodanddrink/foodanddrinknews/11410674/Heston-Blumenthal-puts-a-stop-to-photos-at-the-dinner-table.html

p. 225 '...under the hashtag #couscousforcomment.': https://www.theguardian.com/technology/2019/jul/13/couscousforcomment-the-hashtag-shaming-instagrammers-who-demand-free-food

p. 226 'The Shed in Dulwich was created with...': https://www.vice.com/en_uk/article/434gqw/i-made-my-shed-the-top-rated-restaurant-on-tripadvisor

Chapter 9

p. 230 'On the back of this, she was offered a book deal.': Powell, J. (2009). *Julie & Julia: My Year of Cooking Dangerously*, Penguin.

p. 237 'In the UK and the US, you can't copyright a recipe.': https://www.cla.co.uk/blog/higher-education/copyright-recipes

p. 238 'The US Copyright Office official stipulation says...': http://scireg.org/us_copyright_registration/fls/fl122.html

p. 239 "Food and art may be related in three different ways": Pollack, M. (1990). Intellectual Property Protection for the Creative Chef, or How to Copyright a Cake: A Modest Proposal. *Cardozo L. Rev.*, 12, 1477.

Food and Social Media: You Are What You Tweet, by Signe Rousseau

Chapter 10

p. 246 '72% of Internet users say they have searched...': Research Center. 2011. Peer-to-peer healthcare

http://www.pewinternet.org/Reports/2011/P2PHealthcare.aspx

https://www.pewinternet.org/2013/01/15/peer-to-peer-health-care/

p. 250 'In addition, we have research looking at #fitspo images...': Tiggemann, M., & Zaccardo, M. (2015). "Exercise to be fit, not skinny": The effect of fitspiration imagery on women's body image. *Body image*, 15, 61–67.

p. 256 '...BJSM social media pages, and most read editorial.': Malhotra, A., Redberg, R. F., & Meier, P. (2017). Saturated fat does not clog the arteries: coronary heart disease is a chronic inflammatory condition, the risk of which can be effectively reduced from healthy lifestyle interventions.

p. 257 'a UK-based cardiologist named Aseem Malhotra...': Malhotra, A. (2013). Saturated fat is not the major issue. *BMJ*, 347, f6340.

p. 257 '...for primary and secondary prevention, respectively.': Matthews, A., Herrett, E., Gasparrini, A., Van Staa, T., Goldacre, B., Smeeth, L., & Bhaskaran, K. (2016). Impact of statin related media coverage on use of statins: interrupted time series analysis with UK primary care data. *bmj*, *353*, i3283.

p. 260   Statistics on food waste:

Defra, 2018. Digest of Waste and Resource Statistics – 2018 Edition. UK Government, London. https://assets.publishing. service.gov.uk/government/uploads/system/uploads/ attachment_data/file/710124/Digest_of_Waste_and_Resource_ Statistics_2018.pdf

WRAP, 2017. Household Food Waste in the UK, 2015 http:// www.wrap.org.uk/sites/files/wrap/Household_food_waste_ in_the_UK_2015_Report.pdf

p. 261   '...the supermarket ASDA in the UK.': Young, W., Russell, S. V., Robinson, C. A., & Barkemeyer, R. (2017). Can social media be a tool for reducing consumers' food waste? A behaviour change experiment by a UK retailer. *Resources, Conservation and Recycling*, *117*, 195–203.

p. 262   Dumpster diving accounts: @thetrashwalker, @anurbanharvester, @cookingwithtrashshow, @dumpsterdelights

Chapter 11

p. 266   'That petition spread on social media...': https://petition. parliament.uk/archived/petitions/106651

p. 266   'That September parliament responded to the petition...': https://www.gov.uk/government/news/soft-drinks-industry-levy-comes-into-effect

p. 267   '...mostly from angry Scots.': https://www.change.org/p/ barrs-soft-drinks-company-hands-off-our-irn-bru-please-dont-change-the-recipe-by-cutting-sugar-for-sweeteners

p. 268   "...that's where our #AdEnough campaign comes in": https:// www.jamieoliver.com/features/weve-adenough-of-junk-food-marketing/

p. 270   'We also have the newly created #BiteBack2030...': https:// www.biteback2030.com/openletter

p. 272   '...can put real pressure on legislators.': https://www.alliance4 usefulevidence.org/assets/Social-Media-and-Public-Policy.pdf

p. 276   '…with approximately 80% accuracy': https://www. pewinternet.org/2018/07/11/public-attitudes-toward-political-engagement-on-social-media/

p. 278   'According to a survey by the Pew Research Centre…': PwC Health Research Institute Social Media "Likes" Healthcare: From Marketing to Social Business. 2012. http://download.pwc.com/ie/pubs/2012_social_media_likes_healthcare.pdf

p. 278   Scroll Free September: https://www.rsph.org.uk/our-work/campaigns/scroll-free-september.html

p. 280   '…a 2019 report by the Scientific Advisory Committee on Nutrition,': https://www.gov.uk/government/publications/saturated-fats-and-health-sacn-report

p. 281   'In an interview with the *Guardian*, Tom Watson claims…': https://www.theguardian.com/lifeandstyle/2018/sep/12/tom-watson-lost-seven-stone-reversed-type-2-diabetes-interview

p. 281   'He writes on his blog…': https://www.tom-watson.com/weekly_update_23

p. 282   'As of April 2019, offenders who take a photo…': https://www.bbc.co.uk/news/uk-47902522

p. 283   'Another successful example is Nicola Thorp…': https://petition.parliament.uk/archived/petitions/129823

p. 283   'There are several reasons why that is…': Steinberg, S. B. (2016). #Advocacy: Social Media Activism's Power to Transform Law. *Ky. LJ*, *105*, 413.

Conclusion:

p. 289   Social Comparison Orientation Scale: Gibbons, F. X., & Buunk, B. P. (1999). Individual differences in social comparison: development of a scale of social comparison orientation. *Journal of personality and social psychology*, *76*(1), 129.
This quiz uses the short version of this scale.

p. 290   '…mindset from competition to compassion.': Vimalakanthan, K., Kelly, A. C., & Trac, S. (2018). From competition to compassion: A caregiving approach to intervening with appearance comparisons. *Body image*, *25*, 148–162.

and

Homan, K. J., & Tylka, T. L. (2015). Self-compassion moderates body comparison and appearance self-worth's inverse relationships with body appreciation. *Body image*, *15*, 1–7.

p. 293   Mindful Eating Questionnaire. Adapted from: Framson, C., Kristal, A. R., Schenk, J. M., Littman, A. J., Zeliadt, S., & Benitez, D. (2009). Development and validation of the mindful eating questionnaire. *Journal of the American Dietetic Association*, *109*(8), 1439–1444.

This quiz uses a condensed version of the questionnaire.

pp. 297–298 Multidimensional Perfectionism Scale. Adapted from: Frost, R. O., Marten, P., Lahart, C., & Rosenblate, R. (1990). The dimensions of perfectionism. *Cognitive therapy and research*, *14*(5), 449–468.

This quiz uses a condensed version of the questionnaire.

Acknowledgements

I'm still slightly confused how this is my third book?! It was a great and exciting challenge to write about a topic that has been a key part of my life for many years. As expected, I have a bunch of people to thank.

Firstly, my fabulous family, who have been through a lot in the year I spent writing this. They are always wonderfully supportive, and although my father didn't really understand social media, I wish he were still here to read this. I miss him every day.

To the entire amazing team at Head of Zeus who once again allowed me to write a book I was so keen to write. Also, to the team at Northbank Talent for believing in me in the first place.

Massive thank yous are needed for all the wonderful people I interviewed and who contributed to this book (in alphabetical order): Alan Flanagan, Anjali Mahto, Becky Excell, Carmen Huter, Cassidy, Charlotte Stirling-Reed, Fab Giovanetti, Izy Hossack, Jenny Rosborough, Joshua Wolrich, Kimberley Wilson, Lauren Armes, Maxine Ali, Michelle Elman, P Phillips, Rachel Hugh, Rebecca, Sara Kiyo Popowa, Tally Rye, Zara, and my anonymous contributors Sasha* and Karl*. All your contributions and insights were so valuable.

Finally, huge thanks to everyone who has decided to follow me on social media – I appreciate how much you trust me and how much interest you show in my work.

Index

About the Author

Pixie Turner is a registered nutritionist (RNutr) and science communicator. Alongside her degrees in biochemistry and nutrition, she also has over 130,000 followers on her 'Pixie Nutrition' social media accounts. Pixie has been featured as a nutrition expert on BBC, Sky and Channel 5, and in publications such as *Red* magazine, *Evening Standard*, *Grazia*, the *Telegraph* and more.

www.pixieturnernutrition.com
@pixienutrition